Trends in Specialization: Tomorrow's Medicine

Trends in Specialization: Tomorrow's Medicine

Donald G. Langsley, M.D. and
James H. Darragh, M.D. FRCPC
Editors

American Board of Medical Specialties
Evanston, Illinois

Other Books Published by the American Board of Medical Specialties

Evaluation of Noncognitive Skills and Clinical Performance, Edited by John S. Lloyd, Ph.D., 1982

Evaluating the Skills of Medical Specialists, Edited by John S. Lloyd, Ph.D., and Donald G. Langsley, M.D., 1983

Oral Examinations in Medical Specialty Board Certification, Edited by John S. Lloyd, Ph.D., 1983

Legal Aspects of Certification and Accreditation, Edited by Donald G. Langsley, M.D., 1983

Computer Applications in the Evaluation of Physician Competence, Edited by John S. Lloyd, Ph.D., 1984

Residency Director's Role in Specialty Certification, Edited by John S. Lloyd, Ph.D., 1985

ISBN: 0-934277-06-0

Library of Congress Number: 85-73107

Design/Typesetting: North Coast Associates.
Printed in the United States of America.

Contents

Introduction

Specialization has led to and been associated with improvements in health care. The primary specialties in medicine were recognized several decades ago; in recent years an increasing number of subspecialties have been identified. The member boards of the American Board of Medical Specialties (ABMS) now certify in more than 70 specialties and subspecialties, The Royal College of Physicians and Surgeons of Canada (RCPSC) in 41. There are continuing pressures for the recognition of new subspecialties.

Concerned about the progressive fragmentation of medicine into more and more medical specialties and subspecialties, in 1983 Dr. T. B. Ferguson, President ABMS 1982-84, invited Dr. L.E. McLeod, President RCPSC 1982-84 to convene a joint conference sponsored by ABMS and RCPSC to discuss the future of specialization in medicine. The conference was held in Chicago on March 20, 1985, attended by 140 medical practitioners, educators and administrators.

The conference also provided the opportunity to compare and contrast the organization of the medical specialties and the health care delivery systems in the U.S. and Canada.

This book is based on the conference. Some of the chapters originated as papers delivered at the conference—other chapters were written for the book. At the conference, each attendee participated in two of ten discussion groups. The summaries from the discussion groups are presented in Chapter 7.

Glossary of Abbreviations

AAMC	Association of American Medical Colleges
ABIM	American Board of Internal Medicine
ABMS	American Board of Medical Specialties
ACGME	Accreditation Council for Graduate Medical Education
AHA	American Hospital Association
AMA	American Medical Association
CFMA	Council for Medical Affairs
CFPC	College of Family Physicians of Canada
CMA	Canadian Medical Association
CMSS	Council of Medical Specialty Societies
COCERT	Committee on Certification, Subcertification and Recertification
CPMQ	Corporation professionnelle des medecins du Quebec
DRG	Diagnosis Related Groups
FMG	foreign medical graduate
FSMB	Federation of State Medical Boards
FTC	Federal Trade Commission
GME	graduate medical education
GMENAC	Graduate Medical Education National Advisory Council
HMO	Health Maintenance Organization
IPA	Independent Practice Association
LCSB	Liaison Committee for Specialty Boards
NBME	National Board of Medical Examiners

PA	Physician Assistant
PPO	Preferred Provider Organization
RCPSC	Royal College of Physicians and Surgeons of Canada
RRC	Residency Review Committees
SOSSUS	Study on Surgical Services in the United States
"the Blues"	Blue Cross and Blue Shield pre-paid medical and hospital insurance plans
Note:	Graduate medical education, the period of specialty residency training after the M.D., is referred to as postgraduate medical education in Canada.

Note on the ABMS

Between 1917 and 1933, the first four medical specialty boards—for ophthalmology, otolaryngology, obstetrics and gynecology, and dermatology—were founded in the U.S. On June 13, 1933, at a conference attended by representatives from the four specialty boards, AHA, AAMC, FSMB, AMA Council on Medical Education and Hospitals, and NBME, it was resolved that:

> the examination and certification of specialists is best carried out by the National Boards (specialty boards) . . . ; second, that the efficacy of these boards will be brought to their best level by the formation of an advisory committee or council created by two delegated representatives from the official specialty boards now in existence or in the process of formation and the other organizations at the meeting.

Thus was created the Advisory Board for Medical Specialties. The Constitution and Bylaws were adopted on February 11, 1934.

After 1934, official recognition of specialty boards in the U.S. was based on compliance with the "Essentials for Approval of Examining Boards in Medical Specialties," a document drafted through collaborative efforts of the Advisory Board and the AMA Council on Medical Education. The original "Essentials" were approved by the AMA House of Delegates in June 1934. The "Essentials" have undergone several revisions, both major and minor, and the most recent (ninth) was adopted in 1983.

In 1948, the relationships between the Advisory Board and the AMA were formalized through the establishment of the Liaison Committee for Specialty Boards (LCSB). The members of the LCSB were representatives of the Advisory Board and the AMA Council on Medical Education.

By 1948, 14 new specialty boards had received approval, bringing the total number to 18. Between 1949 and 1969 no new boards were approved by the LCSB. In the next decade (1969-1979), the remaining five specialty boards were approved, bringing the current total to 23 ABMS member boards.

From 1933 to 1970, the Advisory Board operated as a federation of individual specialty boards with a part-time secretary-treasurer. The Articles of Incorporation of the Advisory Board were amended on April 10, 1970, to form the American Board of Medical Specialties (ABMS) with a full-time executive director and headquarters in Evanston, Illinois.

After 1970 there was continuing growth of ABMS. While maintaining primary interest in the evaluation and certification of physician specialists, the areas of concern and influence of ABMS have increased steadily, particularly in education and research. ABMS has issued policy statements on: certification, recertification, the meaning of "board eligible," delineation of staff privileges, and the relationship between specialty board certification and medical licensure.

For additional information, readers should consult the ABMS annual reports and reference handbooks: latest edition July 1985.

Note on the RCPSC

Founded in 1929 by an act of the Canadian Parliament, the RCPSC is a national body with headquarters in Ottawa that develops standards for medical, laboratory and surgical specialties, accredits specialty training programs and conducts examinations for certificates of qualification (specialty certificates).

Initially two specialty qualifications were offered—Fellowship in General Medicine and Fellowship in General Surgery. In 1937, at the request of the Canadian Medical Association, the RCPSC offered specialty qualifications in seven specialties: dermatology, ophthalmology, otolaryngology, pediatrics, diagnostic radiology, therapeutic radiology and urology. Subsequently additional specialty qualifications were added so that in 1985 the RCPSC offered 41 specialty qualifications in medical, laboratory and surgical specialties.

From 1946 until 1972, examinations were conducted at two levels in most specialties, either for Fellowship or for Certification (Fellowship was the higher qualification). After 1971 the Fellowship examinations were discontinued and a single examination has been conducted for Certification in each specialty. Since 1972, Certificants of the RCPSC have been able to apply for membership in the RCPSC as Fellows.

The RCPSC offered the first certificates of special competence based on prior certification in a primary specialty in 1975; subsequently additional certificates of special competence have become available.

At present the RCPSC has grown to more than 23,000 Fellows of whom more than 18,000 reside in Canada. Most specialist physicians and surgeons in Canada are Fellows of the RCPSC. By 1984, the RCPSC had issued more than 27,000 specialty certificates. In recent years more than 1,000 specialty certificates have been granted annually.

Certificates of the RCPSC are recognized by medical licensing authorities in 9 of the 10 Canadian provinces and the Yukon and the Northwest Territories as specialists in the delivery of health care under the medical care acts of each jurisdiction. The exception is the province of Quebec where the Corporation professionnelle des medecins du Quebec (CPMQ) is the medical licensing authority and in addition grants certification of qualification in 31 specialties. There is close co-operation between the RCPSC and the CPMQ. They hold simultaneous written examinations in 10 specialties and conduct conjoint on-site accreditation surveys of the specialty training programs sponsored by the four university medical schools in the province of Quebec.

The RCPSC is not a licensing authority, nor an educational institute, nor a professional medical association with primary responsibility for the welfare of its members. While its purposes are primarily those of certifying and accrediting specialists' training, it assumes in addition voluntary responsibility for the maintenance of competence of its members. Inevitably, although indirectly, it is concerned with the institutions in which health care is provided and the mechanisms of access to those institutions.

For additional information about the RCPSC, readers should consult:

1. Lewis D S, RCPSC 1920-1960, Montreal: McGill University Press, 1962

2. Andison A W and Robichon, J G, Editors, RCPSC 50th Anniversary, Ottawa, 1979

3. Shephard D A E, RCPSC 1960-1980, Ottawa, 1985

4. RCPSC Annual Report and Reference Handbook; latest edition 1984

Certification of Medical Specialists in the United States and Canada

James H. Darragh, M.D. and Donald G. Langsley, M.D.

The Certification of medical specialists is centuries old—it was well developed in Venice as early as the 14th century.[1] However, the growth of specialty medicine in the U.S. and Canada is a 20th century phenomenon of professionalization.[2]

As we entered the 20th century, there was no organized system in the U.S. or Canada for recognizing doctors as specialists. Eighty-five years later, the 23 ABMS member boards offer more than 70 specialty and subspecialty qualifications and the RCPSC offers 41. If present trends continue, ABMS may recognize more than 100 specialties and subspecialties at the end of the 20th century and the RCPSC more than 50.

There are separate but similar systems for certification of medical specialists in the U.S. and Canada. There is no reciprocity between the two systems although some Canadian doctors hold qualifications from ABMS member boards and some doctors in the U.S. hold RCPSC qualifications.

In general, developments in specialty medicine in the U.S. have been repeated 10 to 15 years later in Canada. This is not surprising since many Canadian doctors take graduate medical training in the U.S. and belong to U.S. professional associations.

One of the most striking differences in the two systems is the way in which they started and developed. In the U.S., as a first step the specialty boards were founded and later a central organization was formed, the ABMS, with the specialty board always retaining considerable autonomy. In Canada, from the beginning there was a central organization, the

RCPSC; over the years multiple specialty qualifications developed within the RCPSC. One of the objectives of the RCPSC is to develop national standards for specialists in Canada.

Specialty Medicine in the U.S.

The dates of founding of the approved specialty boards in the U.S. are listed in Table 1. As the U.S. mobilized its medical forces for the Second World War in 1941, there were 15 specialty boards covering the major divisions of medical practice and, as well, the American Board of Internal Medicine (ABIM) recognized three subspecialties: cardiovascular disease, gastroenterology and pulmonary disease.

As outlined in Table 2, the recognition of subspecialties started by the ABIM in 1941 was followed in the post-war years by other specialty boards. This process reached a peak in the 1970s when the majority of the subspecialties were recognized by certificates of special competence.

In the early days of specialty recognition, there were fairly distinct boundaries between the primary specialties. As more subspecialties were recognized, it was inevitable that the boundaries became less clear and at times there was overlap. Some areas of special competence were common to more than one primary specialty: emergency care, critical care, nuclear medicine, immunology and immunopathology.

In the 1980s, ABMS searched for a new method for recognizing emerging subspecialties. After lengthy debate, ABMS approved a third type of certificate "added qualification" at the March 1985 meeting.

The requirements for certification by the ABMS member boards are listed in Table 3. Each ABMS member board can set its own requirements for general and special certificates. There is marked variation in the requirements of the 23 member boards; preliminary training requirements vary from zero to five years; specialty training requirements from one to five years; and total years to certification (minimum) from three to eight years. All 23 member boards hold written examinations for certification; 16 of the 23 boards hold oral examinations as well.

The general certificates granted by the ABMS member boards from 1975 to 1984 are listed in Table 4. The average number of certificates granted per year is 16,000; this has increased only slightly in the last 10 years. By far the largest number of certificates have been granted by ABIM, followed closely by the American Board of Family Practice (ABFP). Seven of the 23 boards have issued nearly three-quarters of the certificates. Except for allergy and immunology, the examinations are held at least once a year.

The special certificates granted by 11 of the ABMS member boards are listed in Table 5. ABIM offers the largest number of special certificates (11), followed closely by the American Board of Pathology which offers 9. ABIM and the American Board of Pediatrics grant similar certificates in six subspecialty areas. Overlap in subspecialty areas is apparent: hematology is offered by three boards; immunology by four boards; and as a result of the March 1985 decision of ABMS, seven specialty boards will offer a special certificate in critical care.

Specialty Medicine in Canada

The chronological development of specialty medicine in Canada is summarized in Table 6.

When the elected governing body of the RCPSC, the Council, approves the establishment of a specialty qualification, the matter is referred to committees for implementation. This involves the determination of the specialty training requirements, the guidelines for accreditation of special training programs, and the formats of the certification examinations. This is a lengthy process and accounts for some of the delays between the time of approval by Council and the date of the first examinations for new specialty.

As in the U.S., the first subspecialties to be recognized were in laboratory medicine and internal medicine. In the mid-1960s the specialty qualifications in pathology, bacteriology and general pathology were replaced by six specialty qualifications in laboratory medicine: anatomical pathology, general pathology, hematological pathology, medical biochemistry, medical microbiology and neuropathology. As outlined in Table 7, the RCPSC still offers the same specialty qualifications in laboratory medicine 20 years later.

When it came to recognizing subspecialties of internal medicine and pediatrics, the RCPSC did not follow the U.S. system. ABIM required certification in internal medicine as a prerequisite to certification in a subspecialty and so did the American Board of Pediatrics. The RCPSC recognized cardiology, clinical immunology, hematology, gastroenterology, rheumatology and respiratory medicine as primary specialties. Two core years of training in either internal medicine or pediatrics were necessary, but certification in internal medicine or pediatrics was not necessary. Although this decision was taken by the RCPSC Council in the 1960s, the first examinations in some of those specialties were not held until the 1970s.

After the first examinations for the specialty qualifications in the six medical and pediatric specialties listed above, it was realized that this new system weakened the primary qualifications in internal medicine and pediatrics. In the opinions of an increasing number of members of the RCPSC, the ABMS system should have been followed, that is, the basic specialty qualifications in internal medicine or pediatrics should be required before proceeding to certification in cardiology, clinical immunology, hematology, gastroenterology, rheumatology or respiratory medicine.

After extensive consultation with the 16 Canadian medical schools, the RCPSC specialty committees and the national specialty societies, in 1979 the Council approved a "roll-back"—the regulations were changed and by 1985 it became necessary to have a RCPSC specialty qualification in internal medicine or pediatrics before qualifying for a certificate of special competence in one of the medical or pediatric subspecialties. However, some subspecialists resisted the "roll-back," particularly the cardiologists.

As outlined in the notes to Table 6, the names of several RCPSC specialty qualifications have been changed over the years following similar trends in the U.S.

In two instances a specialty qualification was approved by the RCPSC Council only to be rescinded at a later date.

In 1969, the RCPSC Council approved the establishment of a specialty qualification in child psychiatry. Three years later, Council cancelled the specialty qualification in child psychiatry on the recommendation of the Canadian Psychiatric Association and the RCPSC Specialty Committee in Psychiatry.

Reacting to a petition from the Canadian College of Medical Geneticists, in 1979, the RCPSC Council authorized the establishment of a specialty qualification in medical genetics, a certificate of special competence based on primary certification in internal medicine or pediatrics. The Canadian College of Medical Geneticists did not agree with this decision—it requested primary certification in genetics, not a certificate of special competence. After several years the controversy was not resolved, and in 1983, the RCPSC Council rescinded the proposal to establish a specialty qualification in medical genetics.

In addition to the specialties listed in Table 6, two other groups of specialty qualifications should be mentioned: specialty qualifications which have been approved by the RCPSC Council, but for which the first examination has not been held; and those specialties being considered by the committees of the RCPSC at the request of a national specialty society.

There are five specialties in the first category: perinatal medicine (based on primary certification in obstetrics and gynecology); neonatology (based on primary certification in pediatrics); occupational medicine and critical care medicine. Examples of specialties in the latter group are clinical pharmacology, two additional subspecialtes in obstetrics and gynecology (reproductive medicine and gynecological oncology), and surgical oncology.

The specialty qualifications offered by the RCPSC in 1985 are listed in Table 7. There are 29 specialty qualifications in the Division of Medicine and 12 in the Division of Surgery. The former are divided into clinical specialties (23) and laboratory specialties (6). Of the 41 specialty qualifications, 27 are for certification in a "primary" specialty and 14 are for certificates of special competence based on prior certification in one or more of the primary specialties.

A comparison of the lists of specialty qualifications in Table 7 with the list of ABMS certificates in Table 2 reveals many similarities and some differences. The RCPSC offers a specialty qualification in geriatric medicine. This has been discussed by ABMS, but so far no decision has been taken.

Over the years, the RCPSC has devised a system for the establishment of a new specialty qualification. A petition is made to the RCPSC by a specialty group or association for the recognition of a new specialty using the guidelines in Table 8. Drafted in 1974 after a two year moratorium on the recognition of new specialties, the guidelines were modified in 1982 with the addition of the last sentence in guideline No. 6, "There should be emphasis on university involvement and recognition of the discipline."

The petition is referred to a standing committee, originally the Specialties and Manpower Committee and currently the Committee on Specialties. After reviewing the petition and consulting other specialties, the deans of Canadian medical schools and the relevant national specialty societies, the Committee on Specialties may make a recommendation to Council that a specialty qualification be established. If this recommendation is approved by Council, the Executive Committee of the Council appoints a specialty committee to develop the key documents for the new specialty: the specialty training requirements, the specific guidelines for the accreditation of training programs, and the format of the examinations. These documents must be approved by the appropriate standing committees and finally by the Council before the first examinations are announced. It frequently takes five years from the original petition to the time of first examinations for the new specialty.

Certification for a new specialty is by examination; however, in the three years after the first examinations, when there are no RCPSC accredited training programs, candidates are admitted to the examinations on the basis of training in related specialties and experience. In the fourth year after the first examinations, only candidates who have completed training in accredited training programs are admitted to the examinations.

Table 9 summarizes the more than 10,000 certificates of qualification granted by the RCPSC during the 10 year period 1975 to 1984. More certificates have been granted in recent years with the availability of certificates of special competence. Many doctors hold more than one RCPSC specialty qualification. In some specialties, there is only a small number of candidates each year: neuropathology, thoracic surgery and pediatric general surgery.

General Practice, Family Practice and Family Medicine

In the U.S. and Canada there were similar developments in general practice following the Second World War. Many doctors had special training and experience in the armed forces. In the post-war years, there was emphasis on specialty practice, particularly in the large hospitals in urban centers. General practitioners found that their hospital privileges were being eroded. There was emphasis on continuing medical education for specialists and frequently there were not similar opportunities for general practitioners.

Quite naturally general practitioners reacted by forming their own associations to promote medical education, and they attempted to regain their former status in hospitals and other health care facilities. In the U.S., discussions regarding the formation of a certifying board for family practice were started in the 1940s and led eventually to the founding of the American Board of Family Practice in 1969. (See Tables 1, 2, 3 and 5).

In Canada, a similar movement occurred in the late 1940s and early 1950s. The RCPSC formed a committee to advise Council whether the College should establish a specialty qualification for general practice. Adopting the committee's recommendation, Council declined to establish a specialty qualification in general practice. This led to the foundation in 1954 of the College of General Practice of Canada. In 1969, the name was changed to the College of Family Physicians of Canada (CFPC). Certification examinations in family medicine was established with training programs in all 16 Canadian medical schools. The CFPC stressed educational objectives, criterion referenced examinations and continuing medical education.

Accreditation of Training Programs in U.S. and Canada

The development of a new specialty followed a similar pattern in the U.S. and Canada. Informal training programs were started centered on expertise in an area of medicine or surgery or a field of health care delivery. Soon there was a demand to certify the graduates of those programs. To improve the results at the examinations and the quality of graduate medical education, it was necessary to have regulation of training programs by developing standards and periodic accreditation visits.

In the U.S., this led to the formation of Residency Review Committees (RRC) for each specialty. The RRCs report to the ACGME, an organization sponsored by several U.S. national organizations. This accreditation process developed independently of ABMS although sponsored by ABMS and the member boards.

The accreditation process was gradually extended, but it was not until the 1980s that plans were developed for the accreditation of subspecialty training programs.

A similar process occurred in Canada. In the 1940s, the RCPSC formed a committee for the approval of hospitals for residency training. At first, the College relied on survey material obtained by the Canadian Council on Hospital Accreditation. But by the mid-1960s, it was apparent that the RCPSC would have to develop its own accreditation process. In the next 20 years, the accreditation process was gradually refined and developed with periodic on-site visits, generally every five to six years, to each of the 16 Canadian medical schools in rotation. General standards for the accreditation of specialty training programs were published as well as specific guidelines for the accreditation of training programs in each of the specialties. Every July, the RCPSC publishes a book listing the accredited specialty programs in Canada, the program directors, and the participating hospitals. For credentialing, the RCPSC recognizes "equivalent training" taken outside of Canada. The latter is evaluated on the basis of documents; the RCPSC does not conduct accreditation visits outside of Canada.

Initially, the RCPSC accredited hospitals and hospital programs, sometimes for one or two years. Some residents were able to fulfil the specialty training requirements by assembling short periods of training in individual hospitals without having a coordinated program or progressive responsibility. In the 1970s, led by the CPMQ, there was a movement to place all graduate medical education in Canada under the jurisdiction of the university medical schools. This occurred in the province of Quebec in 1970 and the RCPSC adopted the same policy a few years later. The rationale for this drastic step was that some hospitals, even large teaching hospitals, did not have sufficient resources to meet the educational objectives of specialty training programs. The combined resources of a network of hospitals in a university center were necessary, and for some programs, the resources of the university itself.

Recertification

In the early years of certification of medical specialties in U.S. and Canada, the meaning of certification was not clearly established. One interpretation is that certification is like a university degree—it implies a certain standard of knowledge and a degree of competence at a point in time with no definite reference to future performance. Another interpretation is that certification is good for the lifetime of the holder and implies a continuing level of competence and performance.

From its founding in 1969, the American Board of Family Practice established a trend by granting time limited certificates. Certification in family practice is valid for seven years; an evaluation was necessary to renew certification for an additional period. This led to the "maintenance of competence" movement with periodic evaluation of competence and performance.

At its March 1973 Annual Meeting, the ABMS membership took the following action:

> It was moved, seconded and carried that ABMS adopt in principle, and urge concurrence of its member boards with the policy that voluntary, periodic recertification of medical specialists become an integral part of all national medical specialty programs and, further, that ABMS establish a reasonable deadline when voluntary periodic recertification of medical specialists will become a standard policy of all member boards.

At the 1975 Annual Meeting, the ABMS membership adopted guidelines for recertification which were revised in 1980. All 23 primary and conjoint boards now endorse the principle of recertification.

The ABIM held the first recertification examinations in 1974. This was followed by recertification examinations in other specialties as outlined in Table 2.

Canadians watched the recertification movement in the U.S. with interest. Some Canadian doctors with ABIM member board qualifications took the recertification examinations. As of 1985, the RCPSC has not established a policy on recertification.

The Effect of Recognition of Subspecialties on Primary Specialties

While leading to an improvement in health care, the development of specialties and subspecialties has led to profound changes in health care and the practice and teaching of medicine. As well the deliniation of hospital privileges, the allotment of hospital resources and the determination of fee schedules have been influenced by certification in the primary specialties and subspecialties.

Soon after the program for special certificates in the subspecialties was established, it was apparent that each subspecialty certificate decreased the value and importance of the general certificate. This is one of the reasons why only 11 of the 23 ABMS member boards grant special certificates. This led the ABMS to approve the following statement at the 1975 Interim Meeting as part of the policy statement on the significance of certification in medical specialties:

> Many thoughtful observers, both within and outside of the profession, caution that the progressive fragmentation of medicine into more and more medical specialties and subspecialties is contrary to the best interest of the public. Nevertheless, the established specialty boards—as well as the American Board of Medical Specialties itself—increasingly are facing concerted pressures to offer certification in additional specialty or subspecialty categories. This is occuring despite the fact that accredited educational programs and the evaluative examinations on which general certifications as based assign appropriate emphasis to each of the subspecialties—or areas of special competence—identified with the corresponding primary field. Accordingly, diplomates holding general certification normally acquire, to a greater or lesser degree, all of such competencies in their educational and specialty practice experience.
>
> There is no requirement or necessity for a diplomate in a recognized specialty to hold special certification in a subspecialty of that field in order to be considered qualified to include aspects of that subspecialty within a specialty practice. Under no circumstances should a diplomate be considered unqualified to practice within an area of a subspecialty solely because of lack of subspecialty certification.

These were some of the problems addressed in the position papers and by the discussion groups at the conference.

References

1. See Appendix: 1984: Ell S R.
2. See Appendix: 1985: Shephard D A E.

Tables

Table 1. Dates of Founding of the ABMS Member Boards

American Board of Ophthalmology[1]	1917
American Board of Otolaryngology	1924
American Board of Obstetrics and Gynecology	1930
American Board of Dermatology[2]	1932
(Advisory Board for Medical Specialties - 1933)	
American Board of Pediatrics	1933
American Board of Orthopaedic Surgery	1935
American Board of Psychiatry and Neurology	1935
American Board of Radiology	1935
American Board of Urology	1935
American Board of Internal Medicine	1936
American Board of Pathology	1936
American Board of Surgery	1937
American Board of Neurological Surgery	1940
American Board of Anesthesiology	1941
American Board of Plastic Surgery	1941
American Board of Physical Medicine and Rehabilitation	1947
American Board of Colon and Rectal Surgery	1949
American Board of Preventive Medicine	1949
American Board of Family Practice	1969
American Board of Thoracic Surgery	1970
(American Board of Medical Specialties - 1970)	
American Board of Allergy and Immunology[3]	1971
American Board of Nuclear Medicine	1971
American Board of Emergency Medicine[4]	1979

[1]Founded in 1917 as the American Board of Ophthalmic Examinations; name changed in 1933.
[2]Founded as the American Board of Dermatology and Syphilology; name changed in 19xx.
[3]Conjoint Board
[4]Conjoint Board (modified)

Table 1. ABMS Member Boards: Categories of Certification

American Board of	General Certifications	Special Certifications	Dates of Initial Certification of Special Competence	Dates of Initial Recertification Examinations
Allergy & Immunology	Allergy & Immunology	Diagnostic Laboratory Immunology	1986	1977
Anesthesiology	Anesthesiology	Critical Care Medicine		
Colon & Rectal Surgery	Colon & Rectal Surgery			
Dermatology	Dermatology	Dermatopathology	1974	
		Dermatological Immunology/ Diagnostic and Laboratory Immunology		
Emergency Medicine	Emergency Medicine			
Family Practice	Family Practice			1976
Internal Medicine	Internal Medicine	Cardiovascular Disease	1941	1974
		Critical Care Medicine		
		Diagnostic Laboratory Immunology	1986	
		Endocrinology and Metabolism	1972	
		Gastroenterology	1941	
		Hematology	1972	
		Infectious Disease	1972	
		Medical Oncology	1973	
		Nephrology	1972	
		Pulmonary Disease	1941	
		Rheumatology	1972	
Neurological Surgery	Neurological Surgery	Critical Care Medicine		
Nuclear Medicine	Nuclear Medicine	Cooperates with American Board of Pathology and American Board of Radiology in Radioisotopic Pathology and Nuclear Radiology		
Obstetrics & Gynecology	Obstetrics & Gynecology	Critical Care Medicine		1978
		Gynecologic Oncology	1974	
		Maternal & Fetal Medicine	1974	
		Reproductive Endocrinology	1974	
Ophthalmology	Ophthalmology			
Orthopaedic Surgery	Orthopaedic Surgery			1983
Otolaryngology	Otolaryngology			

Pathology	Anatomic & Clin. Path.	Blood Banking	1973	
	Anatomic Pathology	Chemical Pathology	1950	
	Clinical Pathology	Dermatopathology	1974	
		Forensic Pathology	1959	
		Hematology	1952	
		Immunopathology	1983	
		Medical Microbiology	1949	
		Neuropathology	1947	
		Radioisotopic Pathology	1974	
Pediatrics	Pediatrics	Diagnostic Laboratory Immunology	1986	1980
		Pediatric Cardiology	1961	
		Pediatric Critical Care Medicine	1987	
		Pediatric Endocrinology	1978	
		Pediatric Hemato-Oncology	1974	
		Pediatric Nephrology	1974	
		Pediatric Pulmonology	1986	
		Neonatal-Perinatal Medicine	1975	
Physical Medicine & Rehabilitation	Physical Medicine & Rehabilitation			
Plastic Surgery	Plastic Surgery			1977
Preventive Medicine	Aerospace Medicine			
	Occupational Medicine			
	Public Health and General Preventive Medicine			
Psychiatry & Neurology	Psychiatry	Child Psychiatry	1959	
	Neurology	Critical Care Medicine		
	Neurology with Special Qualifications in Child Neurology			
Radiology	Radiology	Nuclear Radiology	1957	
	Diagnostic Radiology			
	Therapeutic Radiology			
Surgery	Surgery			1980
		Pediatric Surgery	1975	1982
		Surgical Critical Care		
		General Vascular Surgery	1982	
Thoracic Surgery	Thoracic Surgery			1984
Urology	Urology			1981

Table 3. ABMS Member Boards: Requirements for Specialty Board Certification

American Board of	GME Years Required to Certification: Preliminary Training Requirements	Specialty Residency Training Requirement	Total Years to Certification (Minimum)[1]	Written Exam	Oral Exam
Allergy & Immunology	3	2	5	YES	NO
Anesthesiology	1	3	4	YES	YES
Colon & Rectal Surgery	5	1	6	YES	YES
Dermatology	1	3	4	YES	NO
Emergency Medicine	1	2	3	YES	YES
Family Practice		3	3	YES	NO
Internal Medicine		3	3	YES	NO
Neurological Surgery	1	5	8	YES	YES
Nuclear Medicine	2	2	4	YES	NO
Obstetrics/Gynecology		4	6	YES	YES
Ophthalmology	1	3	4	YES	YES
Orthopaedic Surgery		5	7	YES	YES
Otolaryngology	1	3	5	YES	YES
Pathology		4	4	YES	NO
Pediatrics		3	3	YES	YES
Physical Med. & Rehab.	1	3	4	YES	YES
Plastic Surgery	3	2	5	YES	YES
Preventive Medicine	3	1	4	YES	NO
Psychiatry & Neurology		4	4	YES	YES
Radiology		4	4	YES	YES
Surgery		5	5	YES	YES
Thoracic Surgery	5	2	7	YES	YES
Urology	2	3	6½	YES	YES

[1]Total may be greater than sum of Preliminary Training Requirements and Specialty Training Requirements due to practice experience requirements or other creditable experience.

Table 4. General Certificates 1975—1984

American Board of	1975	1976	1977	1978	1979	1980	1981	1982	1983	1984	10-Year Total
Allergy and Immunology	286	—	304	—	356	—	232	—	238	—	1,416
Anesthesiology	608	497	507	453	479	342	428	471	578	633	4,996
Colon & Rectal Surgery	31	29	31	42	34	38	*	39	31	39	314
Dermatology	223	271	440	275	258	294	257	279	291	258	2,846
Emergency Medicine	—	—	—	—	—	248	356	571	766	911	2,852
Family Practice	1,709	2,276	3,104	4,952	3,146	2,107	1,992	2,115	2,168	2,331	25,900
Internal Medicine	3,324	3,973	4,207	4,566	4,365	4,459	4,413	4,355	4,564	4,633	42,859
Neurological Surgery	82	179	104	99	103	138	101	151	108	116	1,181
Nuclear Medicine	409	713	50	52	53	57	84	75	83	88	1,664
Obstetrics & Gynecology	768	908	829	421	743	780	1,168	891	927	994	8,429
Ophthalmology	502	749	567	517	536	496	490	501	481	237	5,076
Orthopaedic Surgery	524	524	719	659	521	570	527	319	299	504	5,166
Otolaryngology	282	286	284	303	264	121	298	254	255	223	2,570
Pathology	548	607	709	757	583	485	547	510	497	495	5,738
Pediatrics	1,194	1,161	1,110	1,157	1,547	1,550	1,659	1,360	1,301	1,606	13,645
Physical Medicine & Rehab.	65	68	124	114	139	101	121	134	116	131	1,113
Plastic Surgery	132	167	157	145	160	155	199	142	163	185	1,605
Preventive Medicine	105	90	103	86	90	87	—	102	144	157	964
Psychiatry & Neurology	856	1,399	1,500	1,426	1,614	1,564	1,415	1,306	1,123	1,181	13,384
Radiology	1,193	983	952	853	617	919	876	900	918	880	9,091
Surgery	839	790	954	1,151	1,018	1,081	977	897	911	933	9,551
Thoracic Surgery	141	160	146	154	158	110	131	159	136	135	1,430
Urology	437	493	402	385	334	332	309	280	254	273	3,499
Totals	14,258	16,323	17,303	18,567	17,118	16,034	16,580	15,811	16,352	16,943	165,289

* Exam not given because of change in exam date.

Table 5. ABMS Member Boards: Special Certificates* 1975—1984

American Board of	1975	1976	1977	1978	1979	1980	1981	1982	1983	1984	10-Year Total
ALLERGY & IMMUNOLOGY											
Diagnostic Laboratory Immunology											
ANESTHESIOLOGY											
Critical Care Medicine											
DERMATOLOGY											
Dermatopathology	117	48	57	60	55	51	66	50	30	29	563
INTERNAL MEDICINE											
Cardiovascular Disease	1,052	21	1,015	—	1,100	—	1,265	—	1,226	—	5,679
Critical Care Medicine											
Diagnostic Laboratory Immunology											
Endocrinology & Metabolism	293	—	323	—	261	—	354	—	247	—	1,478
Gastroenterology	450	—	557	—	563	—	666	—	681	—	2,917
Hematology	—	345	—	338	—	323	—	265	—	291	1,562
Infectious Disease	—	131	—	236	—	274	—	303	—	281	1,275
Medical Oncology	375	—	508	—	554	—	646		543	—	2,626
Nephrology	—	339	—	392	—	351	—	386	—	377	1,845
Pulmonary Disease	—	368	—	556	—	689	—	658	—	627	2,898
Rheumatology	—	189	—	263	—	330	—	341	—	346	1,469
NEUROLOGICAL SURGERY											
Critical Care Medicine											
OBSTETRICS AND GYNECOLOGY											
Critical Care Medicine											
Gynecologic Oncology	13	23	28	—	31	14	27	27	25	19	207
Maternal and Fetal Medicine	23	29	37	—	44	27	47	35	42	29	313
Reproductive Endocrinology	15	13	14	—	22	15	33	23	27	28	190

PATHOLOGY											
Blood Banking	28	35	28	40	34	25	39	24	28	29	310
Chemical Pathology	3	17	10	8	10	9	8	6	10	5	86
Dermatopathology	27	46	45	51	50	51	51	52	25	21	419
Forensic Pathology	22	36	22	34	30	21	29	28	26	27	275
Hematology	14	45	27	47	26	40	24	21	47	20	311
Immunopathology									75	31	106
Medical Microbiology	8	9	13	14	14	10	16	11	18	5	118
Neuropathology	29	20	20	15	21	19	20	13	17	11	185
Radioisotopic Pathology	42	27	22	14	7	1	4	—	1	—	118
PEDIATRICS											
Diagnostic Laboratory Immunology											
Pediatric Cardiology	34	—	57	22	71	—	70	—	77	—	331
Pediatric Critical Care Medicine											
Pediatric Endocrinology	—	—	—	219	—	60	—	—	104	—	383
Pediatric Hematology Oncology	—	86	—	134	—	134	—	77	—	88	519
Pediatric Nephrology	—	61	—	—	79	—	—	55	—	—	195
Pediatric Pulmonology											
Neonatal Perinatal Medicine	355	—	236	—	244	—	250	—	261	—	1,346
PSYCHIATRY AND NEUROLOGY											
Child Psychiatry	50	76	96	109	121	107	152	149	128	106	1,094
Critical Care Medicine											
RADIOLOGY											
Nuclear Radiology	21	50	46	89	36	58	77	89	84	51	601
SURGERY											
General Vascular Surgery	—	—	—	—	—	—	—	14	388	143	545
Pediatric Surgery	231	70	24	17	—	41	—	38	—	33	454
Surgical Critical Care											

* Special Certificates (Certificates of Special Competence) are granted by a primary board to designate special competence in a subspecialty field represented by that board. Two or more primary specialties may include two or more similar subspecialty areas using the same title and equivalent standards.

Table 6. RCPSC: Specialty Qualifications 1929–1985

Specialty	Year Approved by Council	First Examinations Fellowship	First Examinations Certification
Internal Medicine[2]	1929	1931	1946
General Surgery	1929	1931	1946
Dermatology[3]	1937	1947	1946
Pediatrics	1937	1947	1946
Radiology[4]	1937		
Diagnostic		1949	1946
Radiation Oncology[5]		1949	1946
Ophthalmology	1937	1947	1946
Otolaryngology	1937	1947	1946
Urology	1937	1947	1946
Neurology	1941	1947	1946
Obstetrics and Gynecology[6]	1941	1947	1946
Anesthesia	1942	1951	1946
Neurology and/or Psychiatry[7]	1944	1947	1946
Physical Medicine and Rehabilitation	1944	1947	1946
Neurosurgery	1945	1947	1946
Pathology and Bacteriology[8]	1945	1947	1946
General Pathology	1945	1968	1969
Plastic Surgery	1946	1952	1947
Thoracic Surgery[9]	1946		1950
Public Health[10]	1947		1950
Cardiovascular Thoracic Surgery		1962	1972
Anatomical Pathology	1965	1968	1968
Cardiology[11]	1965	1970	1972
Medical Biochemistry	1965	1968	1968
Neuropathology	1965	1968	1968
Hematology[11]	1966	1971	1972
Hematological Pathology	1966	1968	1968
Clinical Immunology and Allergy[11,12]	1968	1971	1972
Gastroenterology[11]	1968	1971	1972
Respiratory Medicine[11]	1968		1972
Rheumatology[11]	1970		1972
Nuclear Medicine	1973		1976
Community Medicine[10]	1974		1976
Pediatric General Surgery[13]	1975		1976
Thoracic Surgery[13]	1976		1979
Geriatric Medicine[14]	1977		1981
Nephrology[16]	1977		1983
Emergency Medicine	1980		1983
Infectious Diseases[16]	1980		1983
Vascular Surgery[13]	1980		1983
Medical Oncology[15]	1982		1985
Endocrinology and Metabolism[16]	1982		1985

1. After 1971, the examinations for Fellowship were discontinued; starting in 1972, and thereafter, there was a single examination for certification. An amendment to the RCPSC Bylaws in 1972 permitted Certificants to apply for membership in the RCPSC as Fellows.

2. Originally offered as general medicine.

3. Originally offered as dermatology and syphilology; the name of the specialty qualification was changed in 1955.

4. At first there was a single specialty qualification in diagnostic and therapeutic radiology. In 1949, this was split into separate qualifications in diagnostic and therapeutic radiology.

5. Originally offered as therapeutic radiology; the name of the specialty qualification was changed to radiation oncology in 1975.

6. Starting in 1966, only one specialty qualification in obstrics and gynecology was offered.

7. In 1949, this specialty qualification was split into separate certificates in pathology (name changed to anatomical pathology in 1965) and bacteriology (name changed to medical microbiology in 1966).

8. In 1949, the combined specialty qualification was split into separated certificates in neurology and psychiatry.

9. In 1961, thoracic surgery was merged with cardiovascular surgery to embrace the new specialty designation of cardiovascular thoracic surgery. Later, in 1976 a certificate of special competence in thoracic surgery based on prior RCPSC certification in general surgery was offered.

10. In 1974, public health was merged with community medicine.

11. In 1985, the specialty qualification was changed from certification to a certificate of special competence based on prior certification in internal medicine or pediatrics.

12. Originally offered as clinical immunology.

13. Certificate of special competence based on prior certification in general surgery.

14. Certificate of special competence based on prior certification in internal medicine.

15. Certificate of special competence based on prior certification in internal medicine or hematology.

16. Certificate of special competence based on prior certification in internal medicine or pediatrics.

Table 7. RCPSC: Specialty Qualifications Offered 1985

Division of Medicine (29)

Clinical Specialties (23)	Laboratory Medicine Specialties (6)
Anesthesia	Anatomical Pathology
Cardiology*	General Pathology
Clinical Immunology and Allergy*	Hematological Pathology
Community Medicine	Medical Biochemistry
Dermatology	Medical Microbiology
Diagnostic Radiology	Neuropathology
Emergency Medicine	
Endrocrinology and Metabolism*	
Gastroenterology*	
Geriatric Medicine*	
Hematology*	
Infectious Diseases*	
Internal Medicine	
Medical Oncology*	
Nephrology*	
Neurology	
Nuclear Medicine	
Pediatrics	
Physical Medicine and Rehabilitation	
Psychiatry	
Radiation Oncology	
Respiratory Medicine*	
Rheumatology*	

Division of Surgery (12)

Cardiovascular and Thoracic Surgery
General Surgery
Neurosurgery
Obstetrics and Gynecology
Ophthalmology
Orthopedic Surgery
Otolaryngology
Pediatric General Surgery*
Plastic Surgery
Thoracic Surgery*
Urology
Vascular Surgery*

*Certificate of Special Competence

Table 8. RCPSC: Guidelines for the Recognition of a New Specialty

1. The Royal College will consider recognition of a new specialty or the granting of a certificate of special competence when a substantial deficiency in patient care of Canadians has been identified and it is clear and apparent that the creation of this specialty will help to rectify this deficiency.
2. There should be a body of knowledge separately and specifically identifiable with the new specialty.
3. There should be separate and specific skills or expertise associated with the practice of the specialty. This guideline can be applied readily to the procedural skills of many specialties.
4. The specialty should have encouraged or attracted enough de facto recognition that there exist individuals already possessing the knowledge and skills to practice it.
5. The number of such individuals identifiable at the time of application for the new specialty or anticipated to be identifiable, employable, and needed in the country, should be large enough to provide a corps of these professionals able to sustain training programs, annual scientific meetings and the examination process.
6. Recognition of the specialty should have as one of its important objectives advancement of the science and practice of medicine in that discipline including such matters as development of appropriate training programs, evaluation procedures and the attraction of research funds. There should be emphasis on university involvement and recognition of the discipline.
7. The creation of the specialty should lead to improved specialized health care in Canada.
8. Creation of the new specialty should be reviewed in the light of its effect on the other specialties, the College as a whole and the delivery of specialized health care in the country.
9. Recognition of the specialty in other jurisdictions, particularly the U.S.A. and U.K. would be a positive factor in the decision.
10. Existence of national specialist societies and journals devoted to the discipline would be a positive factor in the decision.
11. A specialty may be recognized if it is overwhelmingly in the public interest even though some of the more specific guidelines are not met.
12. There should be a clearly recognized need for specialists in the new discipline outside the teaching centres as well as within them.

Table 9. U.S. Requirements for Approval of New Types of Certificates

Section 9.4. **New Types of Certification, Modification of Existing Types of Certification, Recertification, or Change in Name.**

(a) Prior approval of ABMS is required if any Regular Member proposes creation of a new type of certification, substantive modification of an existing type of certification, recertification, or change in its name. Intent to submit a proposal for an additional or a new form of certification must be announced to all Member organizations at least one year before the meeting at which the formal proposal will be submitted for a vote. A proposal for such action by a Regular Member may be submitted for a vote. A proposal for such action by a Regular Member may be submitted to the Executive Vice-President at any time. The proposal shall be considered by the Executive Committee and thereafter submitted to a vote of the Members. A proposal for such action by a Regular Member may be approved by this Corporation at any meeting of Members at which a quorum is present by an affirmative two-thirds majority of the votes cast by the Voting Representatives at the meeting, provided that not less than one hundred twenty (120) days prior to the meeting, each Member shall have been given (1) a copy of the proposal, and (2) notice that the proposal will be submitted to a vote of Members at the meeting to be held on the date specified in the notice.

(b) Those requests from Primary Boards for new or modified types of certification which relate to special certificates in limited fields of specialties represented by approved Primary or Conjoint Boards will be forwarded to the Executive Vice-President in the following outline:

(1) Name of proposed special field of certification.
(2) Purpose of the proposed new or modified type of certification.
(3) Documentation of the professional and scientific status of this special field.
 a. The existence of a body of scientific medical knowledge underlying the area which is in large part distinct from, or more detailed than, that of other areas in which certification is offered.
 b. The existence of a group of physicians concentrating their practice in the proposed area, the number of such physicians and the annual rate of increase in the past decade, and their geographic distribution at present.
 c. The existing national societies, the principal interest of which is in the proposed area, with an indication of the distribution of academic degrees held by their members and of the association of the membership with the specialists of medicine.
 d. Numerical and geographic identification of medical school and hospital departments, divisions, or other units in which the principal educational effort is devoted to the area proposed for special certification.
(4) The number and names of institutions providing residency and

other acceptable educational programs in the specialty, the total number of positions available, and the number of trainees completing training annually.

(5) The duration and curiculum of existing programs.

(6) The number and type of additional educational programs that can be developed.

(7) The cost of the required special training.

(8) Outline of the qualifications required of applicants for certification, including:
   a. Possession of an appropriate medical degree or its equivalent.
   b. General certification by an approved primary specialty board.
   c. Completion of specified education and training or experience in the special discipline.

(9) Outline of proposed scope of the evaluation for candidates and a description of the method of evaluation.

(10) Copy of the proposed application form for candidates for certification.

(11) A written statement indicating concurrence or specific grounds for objection from each Primary and Conjoint Board having expressed related interests in certifying in the same field.

(12) A statement projecting the needs for and the effect of the new certification on the existing patterns of specialty practice including the effect on the quality as well as the cost of providing such specialty care.

(c) Those requests from Primary or Conjoint Boards for approval of a recertification procedure will be forwarded to the Executive Vice-President in the following outline:

(1) The designation of the basic discipline, special field, or fields (subspecialties or special qualifications areas) in which recertification is to be offered.

(2) An outline of specific qualifications required of applicants for recertification, including:
   a. Interval or intervals between initial certification and first recertification and between initial recertification and subsequent recertifications.
   b. Special preparatory requirements, e.g. continuing educational requirements, submission of practice profile for medical audit, self-assessment examination, etc.

(3) A statement of the nature and extent of involvement, if any, of specialty society(ies) in preparation for and/or actual recertification process.

(4) An outline of the proposed scope of the recertification procedures for candidates and description of the method of evaluation for recertification.

(5) A copy of the proposed application form for candidates for recertification.

(6) A statement of the manner in which successful candidates for recertification will be recognized.

Table 10. RCPSC: Numbers of Successful Candidates at the Specialty Examinations 1975—1984

	1975	1976	1977	1978	1979	1980	1981	1982	1983	1984	10-Year Totals
DIVISION OF MEDICINE											
Clinical Specialties											
Anesthesia	60	50	50	63	62	70	82	92	91	100	720
Cardiology	20	32	27	35	29	30	40	37	38	44	332
Clinical Immunology and Allergy	5	2	4	5	X	3	5	5	9	4	42
Community Medicine[1]	—	4	1	5	8	15	16	18	16	22	105
Dermatology	17	13	21	20	22	20	12	18	19	15	177
Diagnostic Radiology	71	61	64	48	63	54	57	67	57	63	605
Emergency Medicine	—	—	—	—	—	—	—	—	59	48	107
Gastroenterology	9	13	21	16	11	13	13	9	14	11	130
Geriatric Medicine	—	—	—	—	—	—	5	6	7	6	24
Hematology	12	16	12	11	7	11	8	10	7	9	103
Infectious Diseases	—	—	—	—	—	—	—	—	13	8	21
Internal Medicine	184	200	208	182	189	188	154	179	193	213	1,890
Nephrology	—	—	—	—	—	—	—	—	22	8	30
Neurology	23	24	27	18	24	18	24	23	29	34	244
Nuclear Medicine	—	43	14	5	4	3	12	8	8	9	106
Pediatrics	70	83	79	77	77	74	81	97	89	93	820
Physical Medicine and Rehabilitation	5	5	4	8	14	9	12	13	10	12	92
Psychiatry	93	137	128	110	126	113	107	123	102	129	1,168
Public Health[1]	1	3	2	—	—	—	—	—	—	—	6
Radiation Oncology[2]	—	3	7	7	8	4	8	7	8	9	61
Respiratory Medicine	13	9	10	20	11	20	21	22	16	22	164
Rheumatology	5	10	10	9	10	15	15	15	15	12	116
Therapeutic Radiology[2]	4	X	—	—	—	—	—	—	—	—	4

Laboratory Specialties											
Anatomical Pathology	22	28	25	22	21	28	28	30	22	27	253
General Pathology	14	8	5	13	8	11	8	6	5	7	85
Hematological Pathology	3	6	3	2	4	1	3	4	3	6	35
Medical Biochemistry	3	5	2	4	3	5	2	4	7	X	35
Medical Microbiology	6	9	5	10	10	6	10	7	8	10	81
Neuropathology	2	X	1	2	1	5	2	2	1	1	17
DIVISION OF SURGERY											
Cardiovascular and Thoracic Surgery	15	12	14	13	12	10	11	16	16	18	137
General Surgery	94	89	89	79	85	85	71	59	64	60	775
Neurosurgery	8	6	8	5	5	12	7	11	14	13	89
Obstetrics and Gynecology	59	44	56	65	61	59	50	59	48	38	539
Ophthalmology	25	35	24	53	31	33	32	42	38	48	361
Orthopedic Surgery	47	35	45	38	49	31	38	34	36	50	403
Otolaryngology	18	27	20	23	25	20	21	14	17	18	203
Pediatric General Surgery	—	35	4	3	1	5	X	2	3	X	53
Plastic Surgery	14	15	17	15	14	19	18	18	15	20	165
Thoracic Surgery	—	—	—	—	16	2	8	2	3	4	35
Urology	25	20	22	22	20	15	16	23	20	17	200
Vascular Surgery	—	—	—	—	—	—	—	—	67	23	90
Grand Totals	947	1,082	1,029	1,008	1,031	1,007	997	1,082	1,209	1,231	10,623

— no examination
X no candidate
(1) name of specialty changed from Public Health to Community Medicine
(2) name of specialty changed from Therapeutic Radiology to Radiation Oncology

Today's Health Care System: The Role of Specialization in the U.S.

Bruce E. Spivey, M.D.

Evolution of Specialism in U.S.

Ever since the first specialty was identified in this country—ophthalmology in the 1860s—(although several psychiatric societies were formed earlier) the trend toward specialization has been increasing. Clearly, specialization has become and is expected to continue to be part of the fundamental fabric of the practice of medicine in the U.S. A few statistics should drive this point home. At the end of the 19th century, general practitioners represented about 90% of MDs.[1] At the end of the 20th century, a recent study projects that nearly 100% of physicians expect to be board certified specialists if the annual growth rate (7.2%) of physicians obtaining board certification continues. At the end of 1981, 53.2% of physicians were board certified.[2] Clearly, it is the profession's expectation that medical school graduates are not ready to practice medicine independently. Consequently, further training is expected after the M.D. degree with the clear implication that certification in a specialty will be attempted.

Canada's trend toward specialization seems to be declining with fewer graduates achieving certification.

That specialization could take hold in the U.S. is interesting given the dim view of and low esteem accorded to specialists in the early 1800s.

During these years, specialism in the U.S. was associated with quackery and the "specialized" itinerant healers of Europe who were emigrating to the U.S.[1] Conversely, generalists dominated the medical scene both in numbers and in medical schools, the AMA, etc. Generalists served as the role models for medical students. Despite these factors, specialism did grow.

The first field to identify itself and be considered as a specialty by the profession in the U.S. was ophthalmology in 1861. This can be directly attributed to the invention of the ophthalmoscope which led to a greater understanding of the eye and its structure. Ophthalmology's evolution as a specialty exemplifies the process by which specialism developed and continues to develop in this country: a new advance in science or technology results in a group of individuals gaining a special expertise in a given area. To exchange information, these individuals form an organization. A journal usually appears and membership in the organization becomes an indication of distinction and a recognition of competence and excellence in the given area. By the early 1900s most major specialties had defined themselves in this manner.[1]

While many share the view that the major impetuses for a new specialty or subspecialty are advances in science, knowledge or technology, some consider competition from outsiders as a major impetus for specialization.[3,4]

The evolution of subspecialties followed the same pattern as that of specialties. Subspecialization began in surgical areas about 50 years prior to subspecialization in internal medicine, since surgical procedures lend themselves to a clearer distinction of particular skills. In the 1920s, internal medicine subspecialties grew as a result of major advances in pharmacotherapy and in clinical investigation which resulted in considerable new knowledge.[5]

Subspecialization also has become part of the fundamental fabric of medical practice. In the early to mid 1900s, the general practitioner as the role model of medical students and residents was replaced by the specialists and later, the subspecialists, as role models. Subspecializing had distinct economic advantages, a benefit recognized by the students. Subspecializing carried with it considerable prestige as well. Few department chairmen were generalists. Research grants went to subspecialists. Awards were granted to subspecialists far more often than generalists. The current structures in our medical schools, academic medical centers, and research funding perpetuate this emphasis on subspecialization. Recently, however, there has been a renewed emphasis on and interest in primary care, beginning most notably with the recognition of family practice as a specialty and the approval of its Board in 1969.

Evolution of Certification

In the early 1900s, there was a growing concern about the quality and lack of standards for medical education as well as the lack of standards for specialty practice. Flexner's 1910 report focused on the problems in medical student education and many proprietary medical schools closed as a result. In addition, it became clear that many who claimed they practiced a specialty were unqualified. The First World War illustrated how great the need was for some standards in specialty practice. Fifty one percent of those claiming to be ophthalmologists were found by the military to be unqualified.[4]

Not unexpectedly, the first specialty to organize an examining board was ophthalmology—in 1917. Otolaryngologists followed a few years later in 1924. To bring some order, an Advisory Board of Medical Specialties (changed to ABMS in 1970) was established in 1933 by the AMA Council on Medical Education and Hospitals, AMA specialty sections and the four existing boards. Its function was to serve as a coordinating body, to set general standards for the Boards and to settle jurisdictional disputes.

Several reasons for the establishment of certifying boards in the specialties have been offered. Specialty boards were viewed as a way to improve the quality of medical education and medical practice. Paul Starr, however, suggests that competition from outsiders (non-MD specialists) again was a major reason behind board certificaton. He uses ophthalmology and otolaryngology as examples. Both specialties were experiencing considerable competition from outsiders at the time their Boards were established. He also attributes competiton as the reason for the expansion of boards during the Depression years.[4]

Only examinations in surgery and internal medicine were offered initially until well into the 1940s. In the U.S., boards for internal medicine and surgery were approved in 1936 and 1937, respectively. By 1937, 12 boards existed. From 1949 to 1969, no new boards were formed, although there was considerable activity with special certifications. Since 1969 five new boards have been established making a total of 23 boards today.

Certification continues to be voluntary and generally is not tied to state licensing of physicians. Seven state licensing boards will accept specialty board certification in lieu of their own requirements for licensing. Of these, four require physicians so licensed to confine their practice to their specialty; three offer unlimited licenses.[6]

Evolution of Special Certifications

The first certifications of special competence to be offered were in internal medicine disease subspecialties in 1941: cardiovascular disease, gastroenterology, and pulmonary disease. Certifications of special competence in pathology subspecialties followed starting with neuropathology in 1967. Interestingly, the first certification of special competence in surgery was not offered until 1975—pediatric surgery, which I expect can be attributed to the early establishment of boards in most of the surgical subspecialties.

Today there is increasing pressure for the specialty Boards to offer some sort of certification in additional specialty or subspecialty categories that will recognize added or special competence. This pressure is due in part to the fact that hospitals often base new privileges or renewal of hospital privileges on specialty credentials. Many are concerned that this bases hospital privileges on cognitive measures rather than on performance measures. However. performance measures have been difficult to derive.

ABMS has recently approved an "added qualifications" approach, in recognition of the need to credential individuals in newly evolving areas. This approach is, at the same time, sensitive to the need to avoid unnecessary proliferation of certification, credentials or boards and the need to develop reasonable criteria for new specialties, subspecialties and specialties which cross areas. Not unexpectedly, there have been problems associated with the push for new boards and "added qualifications"—for example, with geriatrics which crosses several specialties or with head and neck surgery which is practiced by three different groups.

United States Health Care System

Our health care delivery system does not lend itself to an easy or simple description. Unlike Canada, we do not have national health insurance. The elderly through Medicare and the poor through Medicaid do have some of their health care costs covered, although the proportion paid by the government seems to be decreasing in real costs and in reduced eligibility. Other population groups, for the most part, have health insurance, financed individually or by employers as an employee benefit. There is, however, a growing group of individuals who have no health insurance.

The predominant wisdom of the moment is that prospective payment DRGs is a superficial issue and that a capitated payment system for governmental programs and a prepaid system will exist for the rest of the century.

What sort of role has specialization played in the delivery of health care in the U.S.? In recognition of the complexities of our health care delivery system, I will limit my discussion of specializations' role to its effects on four of the issues I consider most crucial: access to care, cost of care, quality of care, and what I shall call the social structure of medicine in the U.S.

Access to Care

From the beginning of specialization in this country, patients have had direct access to specialty or subspecialty care. In urban and suburban areas, self-referral to specialists and subspecialists, such as a cardiologist, contact lens specialist or a knee surgeon is customary. Whether this freedom of access will continue is a matter of speculation today.

With the increasing popularity of prepaid health care plans as well as regulated rate plans (PPOs) and with more and more patients enrolling in these plans, such as HMOs, IPAs, and CMPs (competitive medical plans which are similar to HMOs but are not subject to the many federal regulations governing HMOs), the relative freedom in access which patients have had will diminish significantly. Many of these prepaid plans limit direct access to non-primary care specialists or subspecialists. They use a "gatekeeper" approach to care, meaning that a primary care physician or, in some instances, a nonphysician provider sees the patient first to determine whether and to whom a patient should be referred.

Recent government regulations have paved the way for the Medicare population to enroll in HMOs and CMPs. The impact of these regulations on current patient-physician relationships and on the way in which care is delivered in this country will be considerable. In my view, these regulations will cause the greatest fundamental change in the life and practice of physicians in the U.S. in this century and possibly ever. Traditional referral lines will be disrupted forever and groups of physicians will be in tense competition with other groups of physicians. Just think for a moment about the numbers of non-primary care specialists and subspecialists in practice today who rely on direct access and long established relationships with many aged patients for their patient case load. Likewise, with primary care physicians as the gatekeeper, other specialists and subspecialists will probably see only the more complex cases and could become, solely, tertiary care providers. In addition, it will be interesting to see what happens when HMOs begin to have more chronically ill patients as enrollees. To cut the associated costs, will primary care physicians be more reluctant to refer a patient to a specialist or a subspecialist for care?

The adverse effects of excessive numbers of specialists and subspecialists on access to care are also of concern. Many view the proliferation (and oversupply) of specialists and subspecialists as detrimental or limiting since many patients needing primary care are denied access due to the availability of fewer primary care physicians.[1,7,8,9]

Cost of Care

Traditionally, a strong economic incentive to specialize and subspecialize has existed. Board certified specialists and subspecialists have charged more for their services, an action generally acceptable to the insurors who have willingly reimbursed some individual specialists or subspecialists at the higher rate.

A subtle shift is occurring, however, and specialized and subspecialized care is being viewed as often costly and sometimes unjustified. Because of the number of specialists and subspecialists in practice today, the demand for their specialized services is such that many are spending more time providing general care and less time providing specialized care, although they are still receiving higher fees than generalists.

Currently, organized medicine and the government are debating the issue of physician reimbursement. The differentials in payment for cognitive (non-procedural) versus procedural services are receiving much attention. Undoubtedly, this attention will turn to differentials between payment for the same service provided by a board certified specialist or by a non-certified one (a generalist). If fee schedules for certified specialists are instituted, there may be more pressure for effective recertification that is based on performance rather than on cognitive measures. How these issues will be resolved is anyone's guess.

Quality of Care

Specialization and subspecialization can enhance as well as detract from quality care. With the explosion of knowledge, by subspecializing in a certain area, physicians gain expertise and competence and can keep their skills at the cutting edge. Patients generally can be assured that they are benefiting from the latest technology and advances in the given subspecialty area.

Alternatively, if the demand for subspecialty care is less than the supply of subspecialists, quality of care may suffer. This is especially true if a subspecialist does not see enough cases to maintain his proficiency or skills. In addition, unnecessary procedures or services may be provided.

Some hold the opinion as well that the predominance of subspecialists lessens quality by the fragmentation of care. If patients see only subspecialists, no one is responsible for the broad and comprehensive care of the whole patient.

Social Structure of Medicine in the U.S.

For the most part, because of the early separation of physicians into their separate certifying Boards and corresponding strong specialty societies, many U.S. physicians tend to think of and identify themselves as specialists first and as physicians second. The issue of specialization appears early in medical school, if not before. Likewise, specialty identification is a fundamental consideration and concern from midway through medical school (my own specialty of ophthalmology leads the pack in requiring an early decision regarding residency). I personally feel this has resulted in less generically trained and capable medical school graduates.

Elaborate "umbrella" organizations have been established and provide forums for discussion and some decision making. Witness the ABMS, CMSS, ACGME, ACCME, RRCs, etc. The natural tendency for any organization is to guard jealously its autonomy and independence. Decisions tend to be made on parochial bases with great territorial concerns. This fragmentation has not helped us with the public, the government and, especially, with non-physician providers. Other specialties have tended to view the intrusion of non-physician providers as a particular problem or concern solely of that specialty and not as a generic physician concern or problem.

Various specialties seem to draw certain personality types and to take on a separate independent life of their own—almost to the exclusion of other colleagues' concerns. The specialty-specific separateness of the accreditation and certification processes is undoubtedly not the root cause, although it certainly contributes to territorial behavior, interprofessional turf battles. This separateness also does little to help medicine if attempts to articulate a single coherent voice to a hostile external environment.

Specialization is inevitable and necessary as we advance the science of medicine. I do not propose we go back! Our Canadian colleagues seem to have certain advantages in that basic decisions concerning specialization are made within a single organizational structure—the RCPSC. As Canadians wrestle with specialization and possible solutions, their experiences will be most helpful and valuable to us in the U.S.

Conclusion

The U.S.'s health care delivery system is undergoing enormous changes that will have profound effects on specialization and subspecialization. Although I did not mention the proposed changes to the way in which our graduate medical education will be financed, these too will have far reaching effects on the numbers and mix of specialists and subspecialists trained. What the future of specialization/subspecialization is in the U.S. and in Canada and how we, as physicians, can influence that future so as to retain those aspects that are in the best interest of the public, our patients, is a discussion of great importance. And the rest of this program and the workshops should, I hope, begin to define some constructive and feasible plans for action.

References

1. Luce JM and Byyny RL. The evolution of medical specialism. *Perspect Biol Med* 1979; 377-89.
2. Becker ER, Culler S, Ohsfeldt R. Impact of board certification on physician practice characteristics. *J Med Ed* 1985; 60: 9-15.
3. Gritzer G. Occupational specialization in medicine: knowledge and market explanations. *Social Health Care* 1981; 2: 251-83.
4. Starr P. *The Social Transformation of American Medicine.* Basic Books, Inc. New York 1982.
5. Beeson PB. The natural history of medical subspecialties. *Ann Int Med* 1980; 93: 624-6.
6. *ABMS Annual Report & Reference Handbook* 1985.
7. Moss NH. Superspecialization: the trend and its impact on American medicine. *Ann NY Acad Sci* 1971; 184: 165-6.
8. Chase RA. Proliferation of certification in medical specialties: productive or counterproductive. *N. Eng J Med* 1976; 294: 497-9.
9. Petersdorf RG. Internal medicine 1976: consequences of subspecialization and technology. *Ann Int Med* 1976; 84: 92-4.

Today's Health Care System: The Role of Specialization in Canada

Ramsay W. Gunton, M.D.

Canada's national medicare system

Among the important factors which influence the evolution of a health care system are the morbidity of the population, the number, quality, and distribution of health care workers, the stage of technologic development, and the involvement of government. In Canada government involvement progressed from the provision of hospitals for smallpox, cholera, tuberculosis, mental illness, and surveillance programs for the safety of food and later drugs, to a comprehensive national medicare system. The pace of this evolution conformed more closely to that of western European nations than to that of the U.S. The catalyst for this process was the socialist government of the prairie province of Saskatchewan which was in power during the depression and dust-bowl of the 1930s. By 1959 there was in place a national hospital insurance program in which costs were shared equally by the provincial and federal governments and premiums were charged to individuals who could pay, in some provinces. Within a decade simple *hospital* insurance had been expanded to include *medical care* insurance. This was impelled by the recommendations of a Royal Commission[1] which reflected the rising expectations of people that health care is a right not a privilege, by the favorable economic climate of the 1960s, and by election promises. It was resisted by organized medicine, some prescient economists, and some provinces.

Universal medicare in Canada has now been in operation for 15 years and can no longer be designated an "insurance" based system. Premiums remain in only three provinces; costs are now borne by general tax revenues. The originally equal federal contribution has been declining in recent years to the discomfiture of provincial governments which bear the constitutional right and responsibility for health. The system is controlled by provincial departments of health which have become paymasters for hospitals, doctors, programs, internships, and residencies, and have the power to regulate the output of medical schools. There are convincing advantages to the Canadian system and these include universal coverage, no denial of service, no upfront payment requirement. For example, in the hospital in which I work[2] there is a cardiac transplantation program. Despite the high cost of this service the decision to proceed with a transplant is based upon patient need, the availability of a donor organ, and the mutual concurrence of the members of the hospital transplant team. The problems with the system are predictable and familiar: alleged over-utilization by patients because there is no user fee, alleged over-servicing by physicians fuelled by the fee-for-service principle, escalating costs resulting in imposed financial constraints, implicit and explicit rationing of services, fees, beds, and equipment. The redeeming features from a professional perspective are the preservation of freedom of choice by physician and patient, freedom of movement and place of practice (although the latter is threatened in one province), fee-for-service principle of payment, and an "opting out" privilege in some provinces. It is now a political reality that there is no turning back from this system. Conservative governments have been elected nationally and in most Canadian provinces and they have left the current medical care system in place, out of recognition of the fact that substantial reduction of benefits would be politically unacceptable.

Impact of the national medicare system on specialization

Certified specialists are the only legal payees for specialist services with the practical result that certification in a specialty is financially obligatory rather than optional for those wishing to practice a specialty. This reinforces an economic distinction in most provinces between specialists and providers of primary care.

Provincial ministries of health control the global budget of hospitals including the educational component. This means that senior mandarins in these ministries, with varying degrees of enlightenment and benevolence, control the total number of residency positions, influence the allocation of positions among the subspecialties, and sanction or inhibit the development of hospital based specialty services through budgetary control.

There is of course professional input into all of these decisions but sometimes political realities are more compelling than the considered views of the profession or the operation of the free market system.

Role of the RCPSC in specialty medicine

The RCPSC differs from corresponding American institutions in that it combines educational and collegial functions with specialty certification and accreditation for all disciplines. It is as if all the American Colleges, all the Specialty Boards, the ABMS, the CMSS and the ACGME were rolled into one organization. These multiple roles for the RCPSC evolved, they were not originally planned, but the system clearly fits our political geography. It should be noted that the population of all of Canada is equal to just one of the larger states of the U.S., for example New York or California.

Significant advantages are that the RCPSC governing Council has the authority to make all final decisions relating to recognition, certification, and accreditation of specialties and training programs. We are proud of the RCPSC but cannot be smug. Internecine rivalries, confrontations, and rumbles of secession occur and the broader problems of proliferating specialty recognition remain—weakening of the primary specialties, possible adverse economic impact on the RCPSC and society, and the uncertain effect of fragmentation of medical care on the individual.

Development of the Specialties in Canada[3]

Examinations were held initially in only the two Divisions of the RCPSC, Medicine and Surgery, until well into the 1940s. In 1939 the decision was taken that the College become the certifying body for specialists in Canada and this led to the recognition of 19 specialties by 1951.[6] Each of these was controlled by a RCPSC specialty committee which stipulated requirements for training and advised on examinations and accreditation of programs.

The floodgates opened in the 1960s pushed by advancing knowledge and technology; there was mounting pressure to recognize more and more specialties. The RCPSC referred these matters to a new committee, rather whimsically termed the Fragmentation Committee, which later evolved into the Committee on Specialty Development and Manpower.

Criteria were developed for the recognition of new specialties.[5] These included: a separate body of knowledge, distinctive skills, minimal sustaining numbers, specialty societies and journals, community need in addition to teaching hospital desire, and most important of all putative benefit to the health care of Canadians. Among the noteworthy decisions were the splitting of pathology into several divisions, the recognition of the subspecialties in internal medicine as free-standing specialties, the recognition of new science and technology as in nuclear medicine, the recognition of new social and demographic trends as in geriatric medicine, and the recogniton of a distinctive type and location of health care delivery as in emergency medicine. The process of specialty recognition was usually initiated by newly formed national specialty societies supported by strong advocacy of leaders in that field in academic institutions. I might add that, not surprisingly, during my tenure as Chairman of the Specialties and Manpower Committee, I can recall no instance of supporting documents with the applications for recognition of new specialties from deans of medical schools, executive directors of hospitals, or officers of insuring agencies. Dr. Robert Chase[6] in 1976 astutely observed that the process of recognition and then certification acted as its own catalyst. The non-specialists in general practice begin to have doubts about their competence in it. They began to refer both simple and complex problems, diminsh their experience, and re-inforce their incompetence. The super-specialist initially welcomes all such patients, later resents the imposition on his time of simple problems, inappropriate to his talents, and begins to think of the non-specialist as incompetent because of his necessity to refer simple problems.

The RCPSC Council became concerned in the early 1970s by the headlong pace of specialty recognition and called a temporary halt, a moratorium, which interestingly corresponded to a similar event in ABMS. Among the options considered to control or rationalize the specialty recognition problem were: a return to the two primary disciplines internal medicine and general surgery, body-system oriented specialties, and a three-dimensional matrix incorporating age, body system, and route of health care delivery. It was eventually concluded that full retrenchment was impossible, new specialties should be recognized by certificates of special competence[7] requiring certification in a primary specialty followed by additional training and evaluaton in the subspecialty. It might be noted here that the RCPSC's emphasis in awarding certificates of special competence was to recognize "added" competence, whereas the ABMS connotation was "depth." In adopting the certificate of special competence route, it was hoped that the additional administrative load would be diminished by local, that is, institutional in-training evaluation, and that national standards could be maintained by computer-based cognitive testing. Unfortunately neither of these hopes was realized or accepted by the specialty committees which insisted upon traditional evaluative methodologies. The one achievement of the moratorium of the 1970s was a "roll-back" of the free-standing subspecialties of internal medicine as the important parent specialty. The pressure for recognition of new specialties still persists unabated and the RCPSC offer 41 specialty qualifications in 1985.[8]

Role of Specialties in Health Care Delivery

The major and traditional role of a RCPSC certificant is to act as consultant to other physicians. A patient is referred to a consultant usually by a family physician or general practitioner; the consultant provides special diagnostic, therapeutic, or procedural skills to the patient; on completion of the consultants's services, the patient is returned to the care of the referring physician. Many consider this to be the ideal role for the certificant acting as a specialist and as a consultant. There is a strong body of opinion in Canada that in a idealized, perfect medical care delivery system, all individuals would obtain their medical care through a primary care physician who is a family physician or general practitoner and who would act as an intermediary for referral of patients to specialists and secondary care institutions when this is needed.

But the real world is never perfect or ideal. RCPSC certificants do provide primary care. A legitimate definition of primary care implies "first contact" or on-going direct contact between the patient and the provider of medical care. That is the patient approaches the provider directly. The primary care may be provided on an "interval" or "one-time" basis only as for one acute short illness or recurrent short term illnesses, or it may be provided on a continuing basis for health maintenance. When specialists provide primary care of the latter type it ofen involves patients with chronic, complex, and difficult medical problems, e.g., insulin dependent diabetes, complicated rheumatoid arthritis, or chronic renal failure, to mention a few such conditions in these situations, it is more efficient and probably economical for the specialist to make his recommendations and give treatment directly to patients. The resulting close professional relationships may then lead to the provision of non-specialized primary care for interval illnesses. Other reasons for the provision of primary care by specialists include patient demand for the in-depth expertise of the specialist, regional manpower distribution, simple efficiency as in non-surgical ophthalmological practice, and tradition. In some communities in Canada it is traditional that specialists such as internists, pediatricians, and to a lesser extent obstetricians and gynecologists provide primary care which conforms more to the on-going global responsibility for an individual or a family assumed by the discipline of family medicine. This type of care has been defined in reports from the Johnson Foundation as "principal" care. The proportion of such care provided by Canadian specialists is substantial but has not yet been quantified and is probably less than in the United States.

The rise of family medicine in Canada in the past 15 years has been an important influence in Canadian medicine. There is a separate College of Family Physicians of Canada (CFPC) whose certificants are specially trained in family medicine with the specific mandate to provide comprehensive continuing care for the family unit with very strong emphasis on prevention and social medicine. Separate academic departments of family medicine in Canada's 16 medical schools compete successfully for curriculum time with traditional departments, just as graduate training programs in family medicine compete for residency positions in teaching hospitals and in "teaching practices." However certificated family physicians remain a minority among the non-specialist physicians in Canada despite their increasing role and numbers. The alternative route to "general," "family," or "principal care" practice is licensure following a traditional rotating or mixed internship. The adequacy of this training has concerned both licensing bodies and medical educators. Several Canadian provinces have or will require two years post-MD training prior to licensure.

A national study of physician manpower in Canada in 1975 indicated that approximately 50% were specialists and 50% non-specialists, although only about 65% of this latter group were in active general practice. An analysis two years ago indicated that the proportion of Canadian medical graduates achieving certification in a RCPSC specialty had declined from 45% to those graduating in the 1960s to 30% of those graduating in the mid-1970s. The reasons for this decline are not clear but among the posible factors are: the emergence and strength of family medicine, the widely prevalent emphasis on increasing need for primary care physicians, diminished career opportunities in the specialties, and the non-specialist career directions of the ever increasing proportion of medical graduates who are women. There may now be an upward trend again in the 1980s.

Where are we now?

In response to this rhetorical question, for Canada, it is important to point out again the substrate of universal national medicare within which specialized medicine exists and reacts. For the Canadian consumer of health services the freedom of access and economic impunity make it an almost perfect system. For doctors, the "gatekeepers" and dominant profession within the system, the prospect is less perfect, despite the many advantageous features which have been earlier noted. The entrepreneurial spirit which motivates new specialty services and new specialties must prevail not only within local departmental and institutional decision-making processes, but against the bureaucracy of government ministries. Even within our Royal College, decisions concerning training (especially when additional years are recommended) cannot be taken without recognition of the impact on available residency positions. Control over these is no longer the prerogative of the profession, the medical schools, and the hospitals. The argument could be made, as health care economists and, admittedly, most citizens do, that government influence on a service which consumes such a significant percentage of public funds is legitimate. It is clear, however, that a majority of the medical profession in Canada views the intrusion with deep concern. It is recognized that qualitatively similar problems are perceived by the profession in the U.S. "Certificates of Need," DRGs, government sponsored HMOs, represent increasing federal influence on health care delivery. To us, these still appear to be amenable to negotiation and adaptation. They are not as irrevocable as ministerial fiat.

The attitude of the public toward specialists and specialization is in some ways ambivalent. On the one hand local and national pride are freely expressed for outstanding technologic and scientific advances, and for distinguished doctors, but on the other hand there seems to be a fairly prevalent sentiment that medical care is deficient in the wisdom, compassion, and omniscience attributed to the fabled family doctor of yesteryears. If there is an "official" position, it is that primary care or "principal" care should be provided by family physicians. Canadian federal and provincial ministers of health, perhaps in the belief that they echo public sentiment, have said there are too many specialists, ignoring specific deficiencies while emphasizing oversupply revealed by manpower studies. It is of course abdundantly clear that specialist care is expected and sought by a sophisticated public which knows more and more about medical science. Although the traditional route to specialized care is by referral, primary care is provided by specialists.

At present there is no forseeable limit to the number of new specialties which will be presented to the RCPSC for recognition. Technology and science will not stop. The current rules and processes of the RCPSC set out the criteria but do not impose a ceiling on numbers. The moratorium of the 1970-73 provided only a temporary lull and a re-ordering of the subspecialties in internal medicine. A new examination of the problems and a new search for potential solutions is welcome.

Rererences

1. Hall Commission, etc. 1963.
2. University Hospital, University of Western Ontario, London. ON.
3. Gunton, R W, in Andison and Robichen RCPSC, 50th Anniversary Publication, Ottowa, ON, 1979.
4. Table 6, Chapter 1.
5. Table 8, Chapter 1.
6. Chase, *N Eng J Med* 1976, see Appendix A.
7. First RCPSC CSC was pediatric general surgery in 1975—see Table 6, Chapter 1.
8. *See* Table 7, Chapter 1.

Problems in Specialization: The U.S. Perspective

William E. Laupus, M.D.

A glance at the topics in the 10 discussion groups summarized in Chapter 7 will identify the proliferation of specialties and subspecialties and their various effects on the health care scene. While conceding that specialization and subspecialization have contributed enormously to the gains in the capabilities and skills of practitioners caring for patients, many credit the continuing proliferation of specialties with a disproportionate share of the increased cost of health care. As each new specialty or subspecialty group reaches core strength, whatever that number may be, it begins to seek recognition as a select group whose special expertise and extended educational exposure then become the established norms and standards for quality in that specialty. How did this come about?

The Board movement is a relatively recent arrival to the American scene, dating to 1917 when the American Board of Ophthalmic Examiners, now the American Board of Ophthalmology, was incorporated. Otolaryngology was next in 1924, obstetrics and gynecology came on the scene in 1930 and the American Board of Dermatology and followed in 1932. These four boards along with the American Hospital Association, the Council on Medical Education and Hospitals of the AMA,the Association of American Medical Colleges, the Federation of State Medical Boards and the National Board of Medical Examiners agreed to the formation of the Advisory Board for Medical Specialties in 1933.

This advisory board for medical specialties was the predecessor of the American Board of Medical Specialties which emerged when the advisory board was reorganized in 1970.

Between the years of 1933 and 1970 the board certification movement grew stronger with the addition of 15 new specialties and the gradual realization that virtually all new physicians were entertaining the goal of becoming specialists in their "discipline." During these years, too, the existing boards came to greatly affect the preparation and quality of candidates qualifying for certification by their requirements—their educational standards, the length of training in residency, the selection of topics for examination, the methods of examination, and so forth.

At the time of the 1970 reorganization of the ABMS new articles of incorporation established it as a federation of the existing 20 boards. Subsequently, three additional boards have joined in the federation, the last being the American Board of Emergency Medicine in 1979. The definition and the purpose of the ABMS are germane to our discussion.

Definition of the American Board of Medical Specialties

The primary function of the ABMS is to assist its members in their efforts to promote the quality and efficiency of the process of evaluating and certifying physician specialists. As may be appropriate, the ABMS may coordinate, lead, or participate in collective efforts to ends. As may be desired by member boards, the ABMS may serve as their spokesman or represent them in relationships with other organizations. The ABMS serves to provide information to the public, the government, the profession, and especially to its member boards. Underlying these functions, the ABMS has a continuing dedication to assist in promoting the health of the public through activities relating to the education of the physician and the evaluation and recognition of physician qualifications for practice.

Purpose of the American Board of Medical Specialties

The statement of purpose included in the articles of incorporation is:

- To improve the standards of medical care.
- To act as spokesman for all approved specialty boards, as a group.
- To resolve problems encountered among and between specialty boards.
- To deal with the applications for approval of proposed new specialty boards, new types of certification, modification of existing types of certification, and related matters.
- To endeavor to avoid duplication of effort by specialty boards.
- To establish and maintain minimal standards of organization and operation of specialty boards.

From these brief excerpts we can see that the ABMS role and relationship with the constituent Boards resides in processes which improve standards of health care, resolve problems between Boards, and avoid duplication of effort while dealing with the process of evaluating and certifying physician specialties and its supervision.

Of the problems which regularly confront ABMS those associated with recognition of qualified practitioners, particularly in new or previously undeveloped areas within the scope of medical practice, are the most perplexing today. Many situations now affect multiple disciplines—critical care medicine is an extreme example which involves 4–7 primary disciplines, each seeking a mechanism to certify the added competence in critical care medicine which a specialist who is already certified in the primary discipline has gained through critical care fellowship training. Critical care medicine after six years is not yet on the track and remains a concern to its sponsors and to the ABMS leadership which has devoted major attention to the problem.

An extension of the critical care type of problem has been the seeking of mechanisms for recognizing additional increments of training, short of a two year fellowship experience, but consistent with acquisition of new skills over a 6-12 month period. Various considerations have been suggested, of which the most promising are certificates of added qualifications and certificates of added educational qualifications.

The so-called territorial or "turf" issues are always serious problems for the ABMS. Vascular surgery was a particular problem among the surgical Boards, a problem which has only recently been resolved. The American Board of Otolaryngology, following the lead of its Academy, has sought recognition of the addition of "head and neck surgery" to its name. Opposition from the American Boards of Surgery, Plastic Surgery, and Thoracic Surgery was inevitable and strong. To date the Academy continues to use head and neck surgery in its name, whereas, the Board's request to follow suit has not gained ABMS approval. Another unresolved territorial area is that of hand surgery, a field which involves the orthopaedic, plastic and surgery boards. After three years of intermittent negotiation, there is little progress and no solution acceptable to the three participating groups of surgical specialists.

Another uncertainty involves the duration of certification—certificates were originally issued for the lifetime of the physician. As more and more groups questioned the appropriateness of certification for an unlimited time, for life, Board programs involving voluntary recertification were begun—all were resoundingly unpopular and poorly supported. Time-limited certification and periodic recertification, the choice of family practice appears to have worked out well. More action from non-medical sources is to be expected in this portion of our responsibilities as competiton increases and certification becomes even more important in defining quality and excellence in the future. The final concern is that of cost additions to the graduate medical education training programs through changes in requirement which lengthen the training period and increase the cost of graduate medical education to the hospital. Our records indicate that member boards of the ABMS have extended training requirement 14 times, including six instances in 1984 and one already in 1985. The AAMC has, in fact, proposed a change in the ABMS by-laws to limit this practice because of its effect upon hospital costs—the Boards counter reaction is one of concern that cost concerns will drive graduate medical education instead of principles more closely related to the body of knowledge and the time required to master it. Suggestions for solution of obvious differences include the use of an *effective impact statement* and open hearings on impact by COCERT where peer considerations could be expressed and could influence outcome short of a voting process which devalues the critical autonomy of the Board in setting the standards which define quality in the specialty.

The ABMS has a role in working out solutions to problems which arise in the process of overseeing the certification process of the constituent Boards. The rapidly changing knowledge base and the impact of new knowledge and new technology have promoted the emergence of new specialty groupings clamoring for recognition. In the process of adjusting to these forces, the structure of certification is threatened by fragmentation of the primary discipline itself and by changes in the marketplace which challenge the very concept of the academic health center.

Problems in Specialization: The Canadian Perspective

Jean G. Couture, M.D.

This chapter concerns the Canadian viewpoint on the problems resulting from the proliferation of specialties. There is probably no doubt in anyone's mind that, with the advancement of medical science, the development of new technology and the identification of an increasing number of new specialties, *there have been significant improvements in health care*. Since these improvements have been remarkable, we can convince ourselves quite easily that the present system works well and does not require too many changes. However, as we will see, some of the problems facing doctors, educators, and administrators can influence the quality of care and endanger the realization of our common objective. This question will be discussed under the following headings: first, an attempt to describe the changes affecting the practicing specialist, the teaching institution, and the administrators of health care, then a review of some problems related to subspecialization that can affect the public.

Changes in the Practice Patterns of Specialists

The increase in the number of specialties, as one can expect, has resulted in more competition for specialty care, a new specialty usually occupying some of the territory of an established one. The health system in Canada facilitates to an extent, a delienation between specialties, since the fee schedules are generally specific to each. However, some problems arise when fees for the same services differ from one specialty to another. This has not prevented the development of territorial problems, which, although more apparent in community hospitals, are just as important in some urban hospitals, since doctors in basic specialties will be rendering a large number of specialty services until they have to share these with newly-arrived subspecialists. Consequently, conflicts arise when exclusive hospital privileges in some disciplines are being requested by these specialists.

With the increase in the number of certificates of special competence, subspecialty practice has become comcentrated mainly in urban and university centers. In Canada, this trend has been accelerated by the reduction of residency positions in most of the provinces, thus limiting the available manpower resources in many specialties. Consequently, manpower needs in some disciplines have become acute in community centers located outside of the major cities. Accessibility of specialized care is then diminished, as it is not available to a great portion of the population.

Since the modern diagnostic and therapeutic facilities are also concentrated in urban centers, patients are more aware of these possibilities and will consult frequently highly qualified specialists for simple problems, like headaches, mild chest pains, or simple breast lesions.

This has resulted in a marked increase of subspecialty medical services, a corresponding attrition in the primary specialties, and a general erosion of the basic specialties, mainly internal medicine but also general surgery, pediatrics and some others. For instance, the general internist is a rare entity in the urban centers and often in the community hospitals. Also, there has been a decrease in the scope of general surgery, according to a survey done by the Canadian Association of General Surgeons from 1968 to 1978. This study has shown that the rate of general surgical procedures declined by 7.4% during that period. As a result, the practice patterns of general surgeons in Canada have changed slightly: the study would seem to indicate that general surgeons spend more time in their offices and in the hospital out-patient departments, and less in the operating room. We know that other basic specialties have also undergone some changes, which are similar in many respects.

Statistics from the Quebec Health Insurance Plan show that between 1979 and 1983 about 30 to 35% of first contact services were administered by specialists; these changes do not seem to be influenced by the manpower situation since, during that five-year period, there was a substantial increase in the number of general practitioners, while the number of specialists increased only slightly. Whether this indicates a trend towards more competition for primary care is open to discussion.

Changes Affecting the Teaching Institutions

As expected, the establishment of new specialties and subspecialties has, to a large extent, strained the resources in the medical schools and hospitals. In the medical schools, the presence of subspecialties has created the need for programs leading to certification, thus bringing new structures and financial obligations. As a result of this development, there is pressure for the formation of divisions within departments and subsequent pressure from divisions to become departments. This trend increases the administrative complexity of the faculty and the demands for additional resources.

The establishment of additional programs in universities has also increased the competition among disciplines for residency positions, at a time when provincial governments are reducing the number of residency plots; this has created some conflicts among specialties and resulted in the absence of a critical mass in some subspecialties, as noted by survey teams of the RCPSC.

From the point of view of some Canadian medical schools, contacted through the Deans of our 16 institutions, the proliferation of accredited programs leading to certification tends to divert the resources in subspecialties and balkanize the training in all but the largest schools. The smaller schools appear to be disadvantaged by the necessity to mount subspecialty programs in a growing number of fields, thus straining resources which are small compared to the larger medical schools. Some medical schools believe that they have been forced to develop subspecialty programs and I quote one of the deans "not because they were perceived as a public necessity, but because they were felt essential for the medical school to remain competitive."

Many deans in Canada feel that a period of a few years of stability is essential, and that resources should be used to enhance the core areas of basic specialties. Some have also noted that, in a country like Canada where the population is dispersed over a large surface of land, resources should be concentrated: there should be fewer residency training programs, but better ones.

With the increase of subspecialties, it becomes difficult for some medical schools to develop a curriculum which is compatible with their mission to train an undifferentiated physician. In some instances, this fundamental objective is not reflected in the teaching content of a highly specialized staff.

Some medical schools find it difficult to recruit teachers who can show patients as whole human beings and who can teach some general areas of the undergraduate curriculum. Therefore, it is increasingly difficult to provide a balanced clinical experience to undergraduate students and residents in their junior years, especially in internal medicine. Consequently, students develop an approach to patients which is microscopic and fractionated, and tend to perpetuate the principle of subspecialization by a choice of careers based on what they have been exposed to, as most of the teaching at the undergraduate level is done by subspecialists. Thus, in the absence of effective generalists, students do not see role models and are more prone to select careers as subspecialists.

These observations from some of the Canadian medical schools seem to indicate that the graduates of our universities contribute further to the fragmentation of medicine and, as we will see later, do not provide an answer to some public needs. Nonetheless, most schools will agree that subspecialties have contributed significantly to research.

The Costs of Health Care

There is no doubt that subspecialization has contributed to the substantial increase in the costs of health care over the past 10 to 20 years. It is a known fact that the establishment of new specialty programs entails new financial resources not only in the universities but also in the health care facilities. For governments, health care takes too great a part of the gross national product, or the gross domestic product in the case of Canadian provinces.

Of course, as doctors, we share some of the responsibility for the escalation of health care costs, but, the question is, to what degree? Politicians in Canada, and probably also in the U.S., find it convenient to tell the public that the medical profession is largely responsible for this increase. To prove their point, they will say that the costs of medical services have increased much more rapidly than government expenditures. Such figures are meaningless unless the costs of medical services are compared with the total costs of health care. Statistics from two Canadian provinces show that the costs of medical services have increased at a much slower pace. If, as Robert Chase (1975) has said, we have become overqualified and deliver services that can be interpretated as a luxury, we can take some of the blame for it, but not as much as politicians would seem to indicate.

One cannot ignore the additional costs to the RCPSC when new specialties are established: the definition of training requirements, the credentialing, the formation of tests committees, the setting of examinations, the accreditation, the increasing load on the secretariat, the committees involved in these various tasks, and the amount of time and money devoted to the administration of our 41 programs. This might have a negative effect on our main functions, which are training and evaluation. I hope we never see the day when the creation of a bureaucratic monstrosity will bring about a decline in our educational functions.

The Public Needs: Remaining Challenges

Although we can be very proud of the fact that the development of new specialties has resulted in significant improvements of medical care, it is not certain that this has been accompanied by a better accessibility to the services. Patients frequently complain that they have some difficulty in obtaining the right medical resources. Consequently, there have been changes in the image of medical services as perceived by the public. This question has been asked to Canadians recently by members of a task force on the allocation of health care resources established by the CMA and who just recently presented its report.

In that part of the report dealing with the impact of technology on the physicians, we can read the following: "The image of a medical service based on general practitioners who were viewed as family friends, has given way to one based on hospital specialists who are seen as highly paid engineers dependent on complex technology." If this is really the way the public sees us in Canada, our image needs to be improved. The report suggests that medical schools have a new challenge, "To maintain the kind of new thought and leadership that is needed to produce a sufficient number of well-rounded doctors who are, in the best sense of the word, generalists." Maybe the term "generalists" should be interpreted in a broader sense and include not only general practitioners or graduates of programs in family medicine but also internists, general pediatricians, general surgeons, gynecologists. The changes in some practice patterns noted previously seem to indicate that primary care will be a shared responsibility for years to come, consequently, it would seem logical to take into account the role of basic specialties in assuring the accessibility of primary care services.

Finally, we must ask ourselves if the public needs are served only by disciplines leading to specialty certification. To formulate this question differently, are concerns with the proliferation of specialties responsible for our lack of interest or perhaps our delayed interest in the development of new sectors important to the public: critical care medicine, trauma, geriatric medicine, emergency medicine and many others.

Trauma is a good example and deserves special mention. Data on accident injuries are absolutely staggering; one death in 12 in the U.S. is due to injury and eight million of the people living today will die of injury. Statistics from Canada are somewhat similar and probably worse, according to Charles Burns, past-president of the Trauma Association of Canada. What have we done to improve teaching, research, and patient care in trauma? Very little.

A recent survey carried out in the 16 Canadian medical schools has shown that trauma receives only minimal attention in the undergraduate medical school curriculum and is not a formal part of the training in most residency programs. The situation is similar in the U.S., according to Georges Sheldon in his address as President of the American Association for the Surgery of Trauma last year. The number of trained traumatologists is small and there is very little assurance that an adequate number of well-qualified trauma specialists will be available by the year 2000. These observations on trauma apply also to other sectors of competence where the establishment of programs is felt to be related to the certification process. Geriatric medicine is another example of a sector where the needs of the public should receive more attention: the medical services to the elderly will increase tremendously in the next few years and will be responsible for 34% of hospital services. Are we prepared for such changes? Probably not.

From this discussion, one cannot conclude that trauma or other so-called horizontal disciplines should be recognized as subspecialties leading to certification. It points to the fact, however, that alternatives are probably necessary since we may have reached the point of diminishing returns.

The approach to solutions, from my own perspective, should take into account the following points: first, there seems to be strong support for recommendations that would strengthen the broadly-based specialties and increase the participation of "generalists" in the health care system. Obviously, a clear definition of the term "generalists" is needed.

Secondly, some consideration should be given to the concept that programs can be dissociated from the certification process and that other forms of recognition can be proposed. And finally, in order to improve health care in areas of competence where certification presents problems or is not required, the establishment of programs should take more into account the needs of the public.

Meeting Tomorrow's Manpower Needs: How Do We Get From Here To There?

Arnold S. Relman, M.D.

Manpower problems can be approached in many different ways. The easiest and least controversial is to ask the question, "How many physicians of what kind are we in fact going to have five years from now, 10 years from now, 15 years from now or whatever?" That question, at least in America now, can be fairly accurately answered. Within a very narrow range of uncertainty, we can predict (from what we know about the input into the system) how many physicians are coming out and what the size of the practicing community will be. A number of groups have attempted this exercise: the SOSSUS study in 1975 did a remarkable job for surgery and the surgical specialties. The Association of Professors of Medicine, under Dr. Alvin Tarlov, have done an equally scholarly job for the internists. The GMENAC Committee in 1980 tried to take an overview and they came up with some quantitative predictions which so far seem to have been borne out very closely. GMENAC said that in the United States by the end of this decade, by 1990, we would have about 525,000 actively practicing physicians or about one for every 420 U.S. residents. By the end of the following decade, by the year 2000, GMENAC said the numbers would be approximately 630,000 actively practicing physicians, or about one for every 400 residents, and, said GMENAC, most of those physicians in practice will be specialists. Judging from the input, we are going to have about 70% of our physicians in specialties in the course of the next decade or so. They will be practicing as specialists even if not certified and the Board's figures have, therefore, to be interpreted with some caution. We may have had in 1981 only 53% Board certified specialists, but certainly the numbers of trainees going into the system now are quite different.

It is rather misleading. If you look at the numbers you might argue that the number going into specialty training is closer to 50% if you can call all internists generalists. But the fact of the matter is that roughly two-thirds of all those who enter initial residency training in internal medicine (which is the largest block of residency training programs in America) are either going to leave after one year to go into some other specialty like radiology or anesthesiology or ophthalmology, or are going to complete three years of medical residency and then go on to become subspecialists. So if you start out with 36% of American medical graduates going into internal medicine in Year-1, at the other end you are going to end up with only about 12 or 10% practicing as general primary care internists. If you look at the system in those terms, you come up with a figure of around 70% of our medical graduates being trained in a specialty, and probably going on to practice that specialty.

Another way of looking at the manpower question is: how many, and what kinds of, physicians do we need? That is a much different and a much harder question and nobody agrees on the answer or even how to go about answering the question.

GMENAC said that at the end of this decade we will need about 466,000 physicians. They calculated that figure by estimating how many physicians were required to take care of the perceived and anticipated health care needs of the country. Using that kind of approach, the needs approach, GMENAC came up with a figure of about 466,000 needed in 1990 or about 60,000 to 70.000 less than we will have. So they anticipated a surplus of about 60,000 to 70,000 at the end of this decade and, by the same technique, a surplus of about 130,000 at the end of the next decade—by the year 2000.

Now those GMENAC estimates did not take account of the fact that what some people (including Tarlov and others) are calling "the third component" of medical care in the United States has been growing very rapidly. The "third component" would include HMOs and all sorts of prepaid, organized systems of health care. At present about 7% of the population is enrolled in these systems, but this number is currently increasing at a compound rate of about 10% per annum. Those of you who are interested in compound interest know that such a rate takes you up to big numbers very quickly. Students of the HMO movement, like Paul Elwood and others, are saying that by the year 2000 we are going to have maybe 40 or 50% of the entire American population being taken care of in those kinds of systems. Now the point is that those organized systems use far fewer physicians per population than the private fee-for-service system does.

While recognizing that HMOs have been taking care of a relatively selected population, and therefore, that physician requirements may change in the future, the fact of the matter is that so far they have been using only about one physician per 800 patients, whereas the national average is around one per 400. So the physician excess predicted by GMENAC may turn out to be a very conservative figure.

GMENAC also said that not only were the total numbers going to be excessive but we would have much too high a percentage of specialists. GMENAC said that we did not need anywhere near 70% of our doctors as specialists. We have heard Dr. Gunton tell us that the ratio of specialists to generalists in Canada is almost the inverse of what we have in the U.S. Yet, in Canada, he tells us there is a fairly wide perception that they may have too many specialists. But all of this speculating, I repeat, is based on a perception of need and it assumes that doctors are meant to serve a special social function, which can be estimated. The underlying assumption is that physicians are servants of the public: there are certain needs out there and the number and kinds of doctors ought to conform to the needs of the public.

Now an alternative view of manpower is one taken by economists and lawyers and many other people, namely that health care and the manpower market is an industry, not a social service, and that market forces should be allowed to determine the supply of doctors. This view has been lately receiving powerful support from those who want to see the cost of health care controlled. They think that an increasing supply of physicians will force physicians' fees down and will make physicians more amenable to participating in alternative financial arrangements, like HMOs, which are thought to be very cost effective. This point of view, the market point of view, has also been supported by those who want to see doctors become more available and more consumer oriented, less controlling and less paternalistic. The general sense is that if there are a lot more doctors out there with a lot more economic competition, not only will the doctors' prices come down but doctors will be more eager to please the consumer and will make themselves more available, will provide services in ways that the consumer wants.

A third force supporting the market place approach is the law. In 1975, the United States Supreme Court ruled in a case involving the Virginia Bar Assocation, that the professions, for purposes of antitrust law, were businesses too. Since that time, the Federal Trade Commission has been exerting increasing influence on the behavior of organized medicine. The law now regards medicine in many ways (not completely—the law is schizophrenic about this) as a business. This means that, under the antitrust laws any collective manpower planning in the private sector (except for those decisions and those policies that bear directly on questions of quality and quality control) are illegal. The market must be allowed to play itself out.

Finally, this point of view has received support, I am sorry to say, from responsible senior spokespersons for organized medicine and other major groups representing hospitals and medical education. These leaders are constrained to maintain the status quo by their constituents' parochial concerns, which are often conflicting. Simply to keep a federation together often requires that one not take a strong stand on a controversial issue. Furthermore, leaders in medicine are understandably intimidated by the prospect of FTC action and antitrust suits. Therefore, they defend the marketplace philosophy and resist any suggestion that the numbers and types of physicians should be actively changed or regulated.

Those who take this marketplace view do not see any reason to do anything about the problem, assuming there is a problem. They say that if the supply of manpower ever greatly exceeds demand, the economic signals (namely, reduced fees and reduced salaries) will feed back to would-be medical students and would-be residents in oversupplied specialties and they will stop coming. So their answer to the question of how we get from here to there is "let Adam Smith's invisible hand take care of it."

Those who take the "needs" approach, those who think that we physicians provide social service—that we are not businessmen, that we are not really operating in a free market—advocate some kind of planning. Some believe that planning should be in the private sector, some believe it should be in the public sector, or both.

But since there is no agreement on what the needs are, and since there are now significant legal impediments in the way of private sector action, we have had essentially no action for the past decade which this problem has been very much in the forefront. So it has looked for a long time to what has been going on as if we simply could not get there from here, assuming of course that you knew where we wanted to go.

Now, a new mechanism (call it, if you will, *deus ex machina*) is appearing. The largest payer of the cost of graduate medical education, i.e. the federal government, has become acutely concerned about its open-ended economic liability under the Medicare Pass-through system, in which the direct costs of graduate medical education are simply added to payments for hospital care. As Dr. Laupus has said, it looks as if cost considerations will drive graduate medical education.

I might say that hospital managers and owners are also concerned about the cost of graduate medical education because that is one of the reasons why teaching hospitals are not competitive in this increasingly price sensitive and price competitive market. Medicare contributes about 40% of the operating revenue of teaching hospitals and this probably means that they are paying about the same percentage of the direct and indirect costs of graduate medical education.

Now at the moment in Washington, there is an acute pressure to reduce federal expenditures in all areas of the U.S. domestic economy. There is particularly acute pressure to reduce medicare expenditure because it seems to be open-ended and expanding very rapidly. So Medicare's costs are going to be reduced and the money spent on graduate medical education is one of the obvious targets. As Dr. Michael Whitcob pointed out a year ago in the *New England Journal of Medicine*,[1] this control of Medicare payment for graduate medical education will be achieved by control of the numbers of funded training slots. That is going to be the mechanism of change, and it seems to me very obvious that it is coming. The question is simply, in what form is it going to come. There are all kinds of ideas now circulating around Capitol Hill and the country, all sorts of plans and proposals. I do not know what the ultimate plan will be, but bills are being introduced and it is a safe bet that there will be some sort of federally-mandated regulation of residency training.

For us in the private sector, this prospect is at once a threat and an opportunity. We are, after all, a pluralistic society and our health care system is a pluralistic one. We do not need to anticipate some kind of total bureaucratic fiat. We can anticipate joint participation by the federal government, by the private third-party payers, and by the professions that are presumably representatives of the public. There is an opporunity for collaboration and compromise.

I do not believe the U.S. Congress wants to do the whole thing by itself. I am sure the Congress would welcome initiatives from the private sector. We can, I think, maintain a certain amount of control of our destiny and preserve rationality and fairness and medical good sense in the graduate medical education system if we will only turn our attention from internal problems about new specialties and certification problems, to working with the gathering external forces that are urging a national plan for graduate medical education. That is the challenge and the opportunity.

References

1. Whitcob, M., N Eng J Med 1986.

Summaries from the Discussion Groups

7.1 Effect of Proliferation of Subspecialties on Certification

C. Rollins Hanlon, M.D. and Yves Morin, M.D.

It is not possible to stop specialization for reasons well known. The evolution of specialization has been somewhat similar in U.S.A. and Canada. Specialists limited their practices to a particular field. Then developed formal fellowship training programs. Those training programs developed an accreditation process, and thereafter there was a great push for certification of the graduates of those programs. In the U.S.A., there have been periodic moratoriums on authorizing accreditation of new specialties e.g. 1972-76, but the proliferation of new specialties has been inexorable.

Certification has definite advantages and it is possible that recertification is an important process or even desirable. Hospitals use certification in assigning privileges to some extent. There are also bad effects from super-specialization. It takes clinical material away from the basic discipline. It takes dollars away from the support of the basic discipline from which it was spawned. In Canada, if you take it away from one place you have to give it to another because the aggregate financial pie is restricted.

The differences between the U.S. and the Canadian systems were exhaustively investigated. There are different control mechanisms, for example, on manpower and resource allocation—which are much neater and tidier in the more closed Canadian system than in the U.S. system.

Alternate routes to certification must be considered. Certification with out examination gets a very poor press from practically everybody. Program directors would have trouble being strict in evaluation, or in dealing harshly with evaluation of their trainees. Program directors sometimes are not totally candid about the graduates of their programs; they have a vested interest in seeing that their people show up well.

The cost of processing candidates for certification must also be considered because of the inordinate charges per candidate in some of the specialties. The simple process of oral evaluation has been dropped in some of the specialties because of logistical problems and cost. That seems to be more a pragmatic consideration than a theoretical one. All potentially restrictive practices in the U.S.A., whether with manpower or any other issue, go on under the baleful eye of the Federal Trade Commission (FTC). If you say specialization has an economic component (and everything in this world has), then the FTC will be interested.

There is great difficulty in dropping the unsatisfactory trainee before completion of a training program; most difficult of all is dropping an individual in the middle of a year. That seems to be easier in Canada because it is not as likely to involve the participants in endless, expensive litigation.

7.2 Subspecialization: An Answer to Public Needs?

Melvin A. Glasser and William B. Spaulding, M.D.

The question as to whether subspecialization is an answer to public needs is really equivocal. The general feeling is that subspecialization meets and addresses a public need. They are probably here to stay but in modified form. Some feel the need for a gatekeeper and for care (this is largely so in Canada) to be managed in the U.S.A. through the use of a gatekeeper. There are some reservations about legal liabilities on the part of the family practitioner or the generalist or the gatekeeper, but some feel that this would help a great deal in meeting public need.

On the other hand, when the question comes up about how the public knows how to pick a gatekeeper, or pick a specialist, that gets to be sticky. The general feeling is that the public does not know, that the public does not understand about the qualifications of specialists and certainly of subspecialists, and only the payers of care (either advocates of the public or insurers or large corporations) are aware of the fact that subspecialties and specialties are added cost factors in escalating the costs of health care in the U.S.

It has been pointed out that the system of referral through a family physician in Canada works quite well with the exception that in a couple of instances like dermatology and ophthalmology there often is a direct approach. In the U.S., it has been emphasized again and again that people do not know how to get into the system. They do not know how to use the specialist and the subspecialist and it is only as they find their way through the maze that they can eventually get the kind of care they need. It is stressed by a number of people, that this system of fragmentation may provide good technical care but has real problems and that we lose a personal physician in the process. We get treatment procedures and we get mechanization and we get tests and the patient frequently ends up without the feeling he has a physician who is taking care of his needs as a person.

There are all kinds of changes in the system that are important to the consumer and to the profession. Examples are the development of HMOs in the U.S. and development of paid physicians on hospital staffs and other prepayment arrangements which, in fact, are reducing the use of subspecialties. There is much more attention to the quality of care, to the needs of subspecialties, to the economics of these situations. An illustration in the U.S. is U.S. corporations which are now doing their own insuring. There is somebody who calls up to ascertain whether this kind of a referral is appropriate or what the qualifications are of the person who is to render the care. These are external factors, of course accentuated now through attention to care in what Canada calls Medicare and what the U.S. calls Medicaid.

Nobody is absolved of responsibilty in this. Reference was made to the medical schools which are now stepping up (in the view of most Americans) to their responsibilities to promote full attention to the patient's needs. Early in medical education in many of the schools, students already think like subspecialists rather then general physicians. Medical schools frequently encourage this, particularly since many of the teaching physicians are themselves subspecialists.

This leads to the issues of subspecialties and specialties and quality of care. It was recognized that we already (in the U.S. at least) recognize that there are not enough patients to keep many specialists and many subspecialists reasonably fully engaged in their particular field. Therefore, they are practicing medicine in areas for which they have inadequate experience and for which we as a society have paid a great deal of money. Some are trained as general surgeons and they act as family physicians. It has been pointed out that otolaryngologists do not have enough procedures to keep them competent and they say so, but nobody has put any brakes on training more otolaryngologists.

These issues are comparable in Canada, except that in Canada the government in several of the provinces now is setting goals for the number of training posts to be made available and two of the provinces have set goals of 50% of all the training spots to be for generalists and family physicians, as opposed to the specialties. In many of the other provinces it is not working that way, but what is working is the fact that the government will not pay for a specialist unless he/she is board certified.

The question of added qualifications (a new type of certification) has been reviewed for the subspecialties. Discomfort has been expressed about the question of additional certification and additional costs of subspecialty examinations in either system or, in fact, in Canada or the U.S. where there is increased sensitivity to the cost factors.

The issue of malpractice was brought up in an interesting way in that there is increasing use of subspecialists to protect the specialists from the danger of malpractice suits. A highly qualified subspecialist is asked to state whether this is an appropriate procedure before it is undertaken and, therefore, the specialist is protected. Obstetrics is often cited as one of the areas.

Questions are often raised about restriction of practice and restriction of residency posts. The question is: "Can we plan for a better allocation of slots? Can we plan for a reduction in posts?" In both countries we know there is no question we are facing a surplus of physicians and a particular surplus in certain geographic areas. The organized medical profession in the U.S. seems to be remaining aloof from the question. In Canada there is some attempt to face it by the government and the profession.

The emphasis is placed on cost containment in the U.S. (with the entrance of the HMO and organized prepaid group practices) by reducing costs and increasing the productivity of physicians. If the medical profession and the specialties do not move into the scene and attempt to work through alternate plans with the government decision makers then the decisions would be made without the professionals and without the specialty organizations. It is generally agreed that that might be an unhappy set of circumstances, one would have to say in conclusion that there were no ringing declarations saying, "On to the trenches. Let's move out and participate in it."

7.3 Subspecialization in Teaching vs Community Hospitals

Richard J. Reitemeier, M.D. and James E. Hickey, M.D.

There have been significant differences between the Canadian and the U.S. systems; as well in Canada there are differences among the provinces. For example, the medical profession has moved to begin work with the government in Manitoba, while it is unlikely that such a move will take place in Quebec. The remaining provinces are somewhere in between.

In contrast, in the U.S., we are organizationally fragmented and cannot speak with the common voice. This contrast and the subject of professional interaction with the government is considered of critical importance if specialization is to have any kind of logical direction and control of the numbers and the kinds of specialists.

The driving force for change in control of the medical systems in both countries is recognized as fiscal. In the U.S. this seems to be depending upon market forces with competition as critical, while in Canada the energy for change is through government bureaucracy. Neither system is directed by logical planning for the needs of the people or the needs of the disciplines or even for the acquisition of necessary facilities. The need for and value of physician involvement in the decision making process at governmental level is clear. The potential does exist, and is being used in some areas, for specialists from some of the tertiary care centers reaching out to the rural hospitals and providing specialty services. To the extent that this is effective, such dampens the need to train more specialists.

In the U.S., for most hospitals, the name of the game is survival and therefore to be competitive and attractive to the various agencies and organizations that are shopping for the cheapest rates. The hospital wishes to present itself as capable of supplying all desired services. So it, therefore, has a motive to obtain more specialists and subspecialists. On top of this is the seeming paradox of the special requirements of the various RRCs of the various specialists and subspecialists necessary for continued accreditation of their residency programs.

We worry about the future of the generalist in the current setting and believe that his future is suspect. We ask the question, "What kind of a patient might be admitted to a hospital by a general internist or general pediatrician or a family practitioner in the future?" The effect of the DRGs and the HMOs may make that question moot and these generalists may end up confining their activities mainly to outpatient facilities.

We agreed that no one is planning manpower by consideration of the needs of the public in the U.S., but note that some efforts are beginning in Canada. We are encouraged to hear that for this issue, the RCPSC and CMA are active and cooperating.

7.4 Criteria for Approving a New Subspecialty

William J. Dignam, M.D. and Charles H. Hollenberg, M.D.

Regardless of how one christens it (a new board, a certificate of special competence or an added qualification) when you put a label on a physician you set up the potential for other physicians being excluded from the area of practice that is so labeled. The various mechanisms that are in place for the recognition of these degrees of expertise are somewhat artificial.

There is a very elaborate mechanism for the recognition of a new board as the accrediting agency for a new specialty. Yet the addition of a year to a residency program can be done independently by a board by just notifying the ABMS that it is taking place. If a physician wishes to add a year to a residency program, he can have that year in an area of subspecialization and, in fact, create a subspecialty. The variety of mechanisms that are in place are perhaps illogical and there is some merit to thinking about having some mechanism for the scrutiny of any suggestion for a new label for a physician.

The relative merits for a single authoritative body (i.e. the RCPSC) in Canada are often cited. Among other things, Canada had the great good sense to have the RCPSC in place before their specialty groups and residency programs came along so that the authority of that group was seldom challenged as might be the case today. There has been a remarkable contribution by the RCPSC since 1972 when the residency programs were all allocated to the 16 Canadian medical schools and were accredited by the RCPSC. This has improved the quality of the graduate medical programs.

In Canada, the funding of the residency positions and setting the number of residency posts is a matter of provincial authority guaranteed by the Canadian constitution. The RCPSC does influence the content and the quality of graduate medical education and does the certifying. The individual university medical centers conduct the programs.

In considering the specific mechanisms that are in place to set up and consider criteria for recognition of new specialties, the criteria of the Liaison Committee for Specialty Boards are more elaborate and more specific than the others, but some assessment of the manpower requirements for the subspecialists should be required. Some assessment of the facilities that would be required from a community, an institution, the faculty, the funding, should be provided in considering new credentials. There should be an assessment of the impact of the recognition of a new area on research.

A consideration of the public interest should be a part of the criteria that are required for the consideration of an application for a new subspecialty. How the public interest is represented in the process of review of the application is always under consideration. The representation of emergency medicine held public hearings to obtain such input.

Consideration should include an assessment of the knowledge and competence in the basic area (general specialty) when one is talking about certificates of special competence or other types of subspecialty training. We felt that there was some difference in emphasis between the RCPSC and the ABMS. It seemed to us that the ABMS is going in the direction of putting a label on shorter and shorter periods of education.

7.5 Economics of Subspecialty Education and Certification

Thomas K. Oliver, Jr., M.D. and Donald R. Wilson, M.D.

In addressing the title "the economics of subspecialty education and certification" one cannot limit the consideration to financing of graduate medical education both for specialties and subspecialties. One must look at the economic issues from a broader base, the cost, and the impact.

The curriculum in medical schools in U.S. and Canada is time-limited (generally four years) and hence, if we add to the curriculum the opportunity to have exposure to all of the surgical and medical subspecialties, something has to give in that time frame. While we believe that it is important for students to have exposure to the subspecialties so that they know something about these fields, the cost of doing this is to reduce the time spent in learning general medicine, general pediatrics, general surgery and the general preparation of the physician. By spending time in subspecialties, students may not achieve the level of competence that they should by the time of the MD degree. Furthermore, they may not see models that attract them to general specialties, and they may more likely be seduced by the subspecialties.

A small Canadian school comments that they feel the need to have most if not all of the subspecialties as part of their curriculum, because they are unable to attract really top quality students to graduate medical education if those subspecialties are not there.

How important is the certificate? One aspect is the cost in the certification process itself. In Canada there are a total of 32 pediatric surgeons. Perhaps one or two will come up for certification each year. It costs the RCPSC between $30,000 and $50,000 to develop a certifying process for a new subspecialty. Everybody knows that the pediatric surgeon has been well trained. He practices in one of a handful of children's hospitals in Canada. That is the only place that he can practice. Why does he need a piece of paper? Yet the response is clearly that it is necessary to be assured of his competence.

We asked ourselves for the evidence that subspecialization improves the academic process of education and research. Obstetrics and gynecology has looked at this and the answer is that their three subspecialties have had a negative effect on education and research. The original programs have been patient care oriented and, the graduates of these programs have been so busy providing subspecialty care in their academic departments that they are spending much less time doing research than they did before.

Does subspecialty training improve care? In obstetrics and gynecology again the answer for oncology is clearly "yes" but it is not clear for the other two subspecialties. Everyone in the discussion group agreed whatever the subspecialty, certification provides the opportunity to charge for it.

What is the role of the well prepared generalist (internist, surgeon, or pediatrician) versus the subspecialist in the care of patients. Three pulmonologists in the discussion group focused on that subspecialty. All three agreed that fully 85 to 90% of what a pulmonologist sees and cares for, can be cared for by the well trained generalist. There is a need for the subspecialist in technical procedures and there is a need for the subspecialist to provide tertiary care for which he is well trained. Many came to the conclusion that we are training too many subspecialists and that we should cut back and limit them largely to academic roles, tertiary care centers, and to technical skills.

If one examines the question of certification of the subspecialist and its impact on subspecialists from other disciplines, there is continued demand for credentialing. An example of this will be certification in critical care medicine. Clearly certification in this subspecialty is going to impact on a number of other subspecialties—pulmonology, cardiology, etc. This needs to be spelled out very carefully because it effects training, care, and turf.

With respect to critical care medicine, Canadians are considering accrediting without certifying by letting the surgeon or pediatrician who wants to have more training focused in this area go ahead and get the training but not have a national credential.

Graduate medical education, whether it is subspecialty or general, provides a considerable amount of care that patients might not otherwise receive—particularly poor patients. Our academic health centers tend to be located in blighted areas. Resident labor is still cheap (relatively speaking) and so it is cost effective.

7.6 Territorial Problems Among Subspecialists

Robert B. King, M.D. and Carroll A. Laurin, M.D.

One territorial problem is in the delivery of procedural services. In this context the discussion group generally agreed that if we can develop criteria of training and the acquisition of skills and care which have the patient as the primary focus, general agreement at both the national and the local level might be reached to resolve these issues without excluding anyone who was qualified from the delivery of services once they were appropriately trained and found to give good care. Fulfiling the needs pertinent to the patient without commitment to specific exclusive medical disciplines softens or resolves more procedural territorial disputes.

The second territorial problem was the delivery and the utilization of resources. Here, with limited resources developing in all of our communities and for a wide variety of reasons and in a wide variety of forms, staged regionalization and the elimination of unwarranted duplication of services and expensive resources within a community seemed critical to a resolution of the dilemma.

A third kind of territorial prerogative, guarded now more perhaps than in years past, is personal time. If one looks at time as territory, we can all recognize that it becomes a highly prized element and a personalized preemption. Many physicians no longer wish to commit their lives to medicine on an open ended time frame. They expect more family time and more opportunity to pursue personal interest—hence they protect time and anticipate that others will function in their absence.

The fourth territorial problem, marketing (just on the horizon) is burgeoning both with respect to individuals and institutions. One is reminded of Barnes Hospital, this magnificent edifice one large city block square, 11 stories high, with a marvelous new front. High on the roof a neon sign says "Barnes Hospital." You can see it 50 miles away coming in by plane on a clear evening. One year later, Children's Hospital put up a blue neon sign right next to it that is 15 feet high. As a matter of fact, the six hospitals in that complex now have a joint committee of their boards of trustees which is specifically charged with developing marketing techniques for the Barnes Hospital group throughout the Mississippi, the Missouri, and the Ohio River Valley districts. It is a new era in competition for the market place and territorial prerogatives.

A fifth was community turf. It was noted that each hospital continues to pursue expansionist programs (a complete "medical center" if you will). So many hospitals have in the last two to three decades tried to become all things to all people far in excess of the resources required for patient care in their communities. This kind of territorial prerogative and reduplication of expensive resources needs to have a hard review, primarily at the level of the boards of trustees of these institutions.

A sixth concern simply stated asks whether our gatekeeper phenomena are anti-competitive and whether they enhance or compromise the equality, cost, and distribution of care and predetermine territorial distribution of resources for economic reasons rather than quality care—the care of the patient being secondary to economic demands.

Finally, by way of trying to deal with some of these issues in a constructive fashion, recognizing that none of them will be resolved in an absolute way (for the scene changes), the question was asked, "Should reconciliation resources be developed by the RCPSC in Canada and by the ABMS in the U.S., specifically tailored to resolving through reconciliation, territorial problems at both the national and the local levels?"

A subtitle for the discussion group of "Strategies for Standing on Shifting Sands" was suggested.

7.7 Subspecialties Involving More Than One Primary Specialty

John A. Benson, Jr., M.D. and John H. Duff, M.D.

The topic of established subspecialties involving more than one primary discipline addresses the issue of diplomates of primary boards seeking certificates of special competence.

The discussion group did not reach a consensus on many points, owing more to differences in approach and definition (experience) than to differences in philosophy. But exchanges of information and ideas were valuable. It was devilishly hard to restrict ourselves to the subject.

The discussion group did agree on two examples of overlapping interest, competence in critical care medicine and geriatrics. One cannot appreciate for the U.S. experience that in Canada there is overlapping interest in most of the subspecialties of internal medicine with pediatrics. In Canada in pediatrics the numbers of subspecialists are small (the numbers trained and the numbers needed for practice). Economics were necessary, but backfired. For example, use of ABIM questions in the RCPSC examination in pulmonary disease, which is available to pediatricians, resulted in complaints from candidates because there had been no questions on children. Indeed, on review the questions largely addressed adult conditions so the candidates got their money back.

There also are examples of extensions of expertise in general surgery, for example, vascular surgery, head and neck oncological surgery, and so forth. A model in this country that has functioned very well (but after some growing pains) is dermatopathology, for which the two Boards have an agency that certifies qualified graduates (dermatologists and pathologists) in this field. Other examples exist, and others are anticipated.

The discussion group agreed that the further development of concurrent qualification of new competences across specialties is likely. Perhaps certification of competence in more complex relationships in patient care (for example, critical care medicine) is doomed to disappointment. There are a variety of skills, standards, and modes of application—the latter depending on local resources, the availability of such specialists and intensive care units, and needs in a small community. It may be easier in allergy or dermatopathology than in critical care medicine. Ultimately, certification should be justified by its effectiveness in protecting the patient.

The question asked of our discussion group was whether certification of all these overlapping special competences is necessary. Once criteria for the recognition of a new special area have been met and when acceptable training is available, is certification of overlapping special competences necessary? Given these circumstances, the discussion group generally regarded certification in a new competence to be preferable and, in fact, inevitable, even if not necessary. Certification may improve the standards of accreditation. Each protects against the imperfections of the other. Trainees want recognition comparable to that provided to their peers trained in other special competences and trained in other primary disciplines. Credentials have become imperatives for the local delineation of privileges, such as hospital staff appointments, procedural privileges, and in malpractice courts.

But discomfort remains, as in our group, about the certificate qua certificate. Would not a certificate from the hospital or the program acknowledging satisfactory completion of training in this special competence be sufficient? There was a good deal of debate about that. It is economical for small programs, such as transplantation surgeons and pediatric surgery in Canada perhaps, and there are other reasons. The final conclusion was that such certificates would do no less harm than one offered by a certifying board. A certificate of satisfactory completion of an accredited training experience in a recognized hospital would be just as apt to be used irrationally as a certificate from a certifying board, given the uncontrolled use of either certificate on the outside. Using only a certificate of satisfactorily completed training may still be an option in Canada. In this country competition and malpractice make that seem unlikely, and the ACGME (and the RCPSC) won't accredit training until there is certification of the resulting competence.

The discussion group, or some of the members, despaired the fragmentation and costly processes inherent in providing certificates in these special competences, particularly overlapping one. They felt professional differentiation must stop at some point. We decided one was apt to be damned if you do (colleagues would deplore the fragmentation created), and damned if you do not (because a board would be seen as forsaking its diplomates in a competitive environment). Furthermore, there are risks in adding certifications when the environment for funding graduate medical education is so threatening.

The question was faced as to whether certificates of special competence by overlapping Boards is harmful. It was assumed that undergraduate and graduate medical education were good. A number of deleterious possible outcomes were brought forth. For example, limiting the field through institutional acceptance has already occurred; in many hospitals the certified internist is not allowed to admit patients or write orders in the coronary care unit. In urban and competitive environments such practices are exclusionary, even if motivated by corporate desires to avoid mistakes and malpractice suits. Might the certificate become a virtual permit? Would it serve the self-interests of the specialist group, have monetary benefits, and so forth? These results of the use of certificates have become a fact of life.

The question was asked, how should new subspecialties that gain approval from the RCPSC or ABMS be handled. Various models were put forth. Should all new certificates be issued by existing primary boards? Could conjoint boards (for instance, the American Board of Allergy and Immunology) be replaced by joint committees? The model is the new untested one of diagnostic laboratory immunology across pediatrics, medicine, and allergy and immunology, where one exam and one pass/fail score apply to all of the specialists entering the exam. Another model is each primary board separately using its own certification process. There are three tickets in hematology in the U.S. If the applicant Boards prevail, there could be six in critical care medicine. There are essentially three in nuclear medicine.

A fourth strategy is working through one board where there are half-a-dozen or more boards seeking certification of the same special competence for their diplomates. One board could offer the exam more economically as agent for the others, and issue the certificate to the diplomates of the other participating boards. The American Board of Pathology has long offered subspecialty certificates to the diplomates of other boards. Another option, which fell on deaf ears several years ago, is for ABMS itself to be the certifying agency. Lastly, of course, an option remains to offer the functional certificate following satisfactory completion of accredited training.

We did not try to resolve which model was better than another, except that perhaps the more complex the competence and the arrangements, the more difficult it becomes to assemble a number of satisfied boards in the conjoint process.

Finally, should there be central control over the issuance of new certificates of special competence involving more than one primary specialty? That seemed logical and it seems to exist in the RCPSC. In the U.S. the individual board has demanded autonomy over standard-setting for the specialists in its discipline. So central control or certification by ABMS do not go down very well with members of the ABMS, but it is certainly logical. If there were central control or if one board permitted another board to examine its diplomates in a new special competence, some relinquishing of autonomy over setting standards would be necessary.

7.8 The Validity of Subspecialty Certification

Henry J. Mankin, M.D. and G. Ross Langley, M.D.

In discussing the validity of subspecialty certification the principal problem is interpretation of the word "validity." Validity, in the generic sense of the entire process of subspecialty certification, was what educators hope we will solve. The discussion group limited itself to validity in the narrow sense (as determined by psychometric techniqes) as applied to certification in subspecialty areas.

There are four parts to the certification procedure for specialties, subspecialties and even for certificates of added qualifications or whatever they are termed:

- first, an educational experience which is sanctioned by a RRC or the RCPSC, and which contains a body of information and a clinical experience of a specified length of time.
- second, a critical review of the performance of an individual by a training chief or faculty.
- third, a practice requirement exists for some boards in the United States.
- fourth, some form of assessment of terminal behavior (usually an examination) which ought to have as an essential feature a test of the validity of the examination.

The group discussed mechanisms of validity and methods of assessment and decided that there were two crucial forms of validity which had to be evaluated if the examination is to be considered valid.

The first form of validity is content validity (defined as a measure of certainty that the material which is used for testing is relevant). And in terms of a subspecialty this implies that the field is well defined and has a finite body of information.

The second form is criterion-related validity which can either be defined as concurrent or predictive. This measurement assesses the value of our testing instrument against some other forms of evaluationary systems (either present or future). So the purpose is to determine if the results of our test are valid when tested against other assessment instruments or can predict the future performance in the "real world."

Turning to the problems of the existence of a subspecialty (a different concept from the term "validity") the group reviewed what we thought were important issues related to establishing the subspecialty as a real discipline. We decided that there were essentially six characteristics thought to be crucial.

The first is that there be a finite body of cognitive information which is related to the core knowledge about the basic specialty and which is specific and has some unique properties. The second characteristic is that there be some psychomotor activity which also is specific and, if not unique, at least clearly related to that subspecialty. The third is a nebulous one (as it has been in our minds since the words were first devised) and that is that there be some aspects of the affective domain which relate to the education of the subspecialist.

Now the next three were tests of the identification of the subspecialty and we think that they are quite important. The first of these is whether the existence of the subspecialty makes the world a better place. Does it make it a better place for care? Does it make it a better place for education? Does it make it a better place for research? Those are hard questions because it is very easy to say "yes" to all of them without much thought, but if looked at carefully it often becomes a little less clear.

The second of these testing questions (which is the fifth characteristic) is, what is the price? What do we have to pay for this? Would it devitalize the parent specialty from which is springs? In a life of limited resources in U.S. and Canada; in a world where so many things require not only our money but our personnel, our time—the most precious commodity of all—what price must we pay for this existence of the subspecialty?

The final one is: Will the subspecialty endure? Will it in three years from now or five years from now, be a "real" discipline? To this point we discussed an example of a major subspecialty of medicine which did not endure, but died for a very good reason (the best reason of all). The subspecialty of pthisiology (those of you who are old enough to remember . . . that it relates to the treatment of tuberculosis) which had all of the characteristics listed above. It had a finite, specific, and quite unique body of cognitive information that was part of the core. There were specific psychomotor activities associated with the subspecialty and the affective domain was important in that it involved the care of chronically ill patients. It clearly made the world a better place and the price was small. The specialty however, did not endure because it "researched itself out of business"; and that is a most desirable way for a subspecialty to serve its public and the parent specialty best.

7.9 Recertification

B. Leslie Huffman, M.D. and Bernard J. Perey, M.D.

Presently 13 U.S. boards have adopted some type of recertification process. Eight of these who are issuing time-limited certificates. These are largely procedure-oriented specialties. Eight of the primary boards have no plans for any recertification process at this point in time. Five of those, however, did endorse the concept of recertification.

The American Board of Family Practice is a pioneer in the field of recertification. The board, founded in 1969, decided from the beginning to have a time-limited certificate of seven years with recertification. Admission to the recertification examination requires having completed continuing medical education and a self-generated review of patient records. In preparation for the examination each candidate selects four topics from a list of 20 different diseases or problems and submits five of his own records for each topic. These are compared to a set of criteria and graded by a computer, which is the state-of-the-art today. In addition to a half day cognitive examination which is a modular exam where three out of six different modules are chosen by the candidate.

The recertification process of the American Board of Obstetrics & Gynecology was discussed at great length. It requires a six months' case list and a personal practice review. This measures both process and outcome. Starting next year Ob/Gyn will go to a time-limited certificate as a mandatory process. The two major purposes of the examination are education and identification of incompetent practitioners.

In Canada there is no formal recertification process with the exception of family medicine. On the other hand, some of the Provinces have such extensive reviews of the clinical practice of physicians that the results are probably as valid as those of any U.S. recertification program. For instance, in the province of Quebec, the activities of physicians are reviewed by professional inspection teams of medical surveyors in each hospital every seven years. The practice of individual physicians functioning outside of hospitals is also reviewed systematically with special attention being given to "high-risk" practitioners. An interesting aspect of these various on-site reviews is that they are carried out by mixed teams of full time surveyors and medical consultants. All these activities are conducted by the licensing authorities. Consequently they may prescribe remedial training for the physician once he has been identified as having shortcomings.

The other recertification going on in Canada is the program of the College of Family Physicians of Canada known as "maintenance of certification." It is adapted to the physician's practice profile. A pre-test is devised on the basis of 200 submitted case histories and is administered. A prescription for learning is written for this physician and then, a post-test is subsequently administered. Interestingly enough, certificates will be withdrawn for failure to participate but not for failure to pass the post-test.

Trainees in residency programs want to know where they stand. They expect to be examined. The consensus in our discussion group was that recertification is not losing its momentum and that there will be increasing demand for it in the future. A member of the group stated emphatically that licensure and certification are a hoax on the public if we do not follow up with recertification. There was some support for this position.

It was our feeling that hospitals will increasingly require recertification from their staff members in order to maintain their privileges. All participants felt that recertification should not be limited to cognitive tests and should include a review of clinical practice (performance). We also all recognized that it is almost impossible to eliminate incompetence with a measure that is voluntary.

7.10 Third Party Payment and Corporatization: Does It Affect Quality?

Fred W. DuVal, M.D. and Kenneth L. Krabbenhoft, M.D.

The groups accepted the definition that a standard is something established by authority, custom, or general consent as a model or example to which similar things should conform. It was also defined as a conspicuous object carried at the top of a pole used as a rallying point, particularly in battle, and that has some relevance. When changes in fee payment are suggested anywhere, the question of standards usually rises.

There was some consensus that accessibility to care was really a portion of quality of care. Ready access to care may improve quality of care. Delays of access, for reasons of third party payment or corporatization, may adversely affect quality of care. That was rather an extension of most concepts of the standard of care.

During the day, the group roamed through the capitation systems, HMOs, the Blues, DRGs, fee-for-service, systems, and the initials of the week—CMP. They are still just initials but both sides came to understand the differences that were going on in Canada's and in U.S.A.'s medical care systems.

The one thing agreed on is that we have a serious defect in that we have no clear criteria for assessing quality of care. Peer review is a little bit like the shifting sands that were referred to earlier and it does not provide you with benchmarks that you may use from decade to decade or year to year, so that we feel that it may not be possible and it may be why there is a dearth of literature on the subject of the quality of care related to the payment system. There may be so many variables in the equation that they cannot be determined.

It was felt that societal and environmental effects of practice currently may be more important to people entering the system (the individuals) than the relative income. And we felt that we need to address or enunciate ways of measuring the quality of care and along with that develop comparable benchmarks that could tell us what is happening to care as it is delivered.

One of the things that was suggested, and I think some of our sociologists are toying with it now, is a realistic measureable "quality of life index." That has such an enchanting title but apparently there is some work being done on quality of life which could be interpreted as, or make some imprints in, reference to the quality of care being delivered. We can all use perinatal death rates, mortality rates, days lost from work—these indices are all used as criteria—but we do not feel that any of them really offer a comparative base that one could use.

Trends in Specialization: Tomorrow's Medicine

Donald G. Langsley, M.D. and James H. Darragh, M.D.

History and geography have given the U.S. and Canada many common features in their medical care systems. Though there are differences, such as a higher level of government control in Canada, the common language and comparable standards of medical education make the emphasis on specialization very similar. Indeed, some Canadians come to the U.S. for specialty education and belong to U.S.-based specialty societies. In like fashion, U.S. citizens sometimes go to Canada for medical school and for graduate medical education. The training for internists or surgeons are similar in both countries; the systems of accrediting training programs or certifying specialists/subspecialists have much in common.

There are differences: in Canada the RCPSC is responsible for *both* accreditation and certification of all specialties except family practice, a separate college represented by the College of Family Physicians of Canada; the U.S. has separate organizations and systems for certification and accreditation. Canada's population is approximately one-tenth that of the U.S. Perhaps the size, as well as history, has enabled Canada to keep all of its graduate medical education within the medical schools. To the U.S. medical educator, keeping track of only 16 medical schools (and thus no more than 16 residency programs in any specialty) seems highly desirable when one realizes that there are 127 medical schools in the U.S. and as many as 430 separate residencies in one specialty (e.g. internal medicine). Canadians do not have the separation of medical schools or academic medical centers from community based teaching hospitals which is common in the U.S.

Nevertheless, the two countries share many similar concerns, as is evident from the chapters of this book and the reports of discussion groups (chapter 7).

In both countries, there is agreement that the impact of certification has been a major influence on the organization of health care. Though there is little *hard* data to demonstrate that certification has improved the quality of health care, this is the conviction of all professionals, and the public. People seek specialists for complex illnesses. Though an article of faith rather than proven fact, the certification process has "driven" the system of specialist education, the use of hospital privileges to control what a physician is permitted to do in the hospital, and the organization of group practices which are frequently multi-specialty in nature. The certification process has also altered the role of professional associations since the specialist is more apt to identify with his specialty or subspecialty than with the general, broad field of medicine. This shows itself in the different roles of the specialty societies and the national medical associations such as the AMA and the CMA.

As pointed out in Chapter 1, a major difference in the history of certification in Canada and the U.S. is that in Canada, certification and accreditation in *all* specialties (except family practice) has been under the aegis of a single organization (the RCPSC). This has permitted a uniformity of standards for training and examination across specialties. In the U.S., the two functions of certification and accreditation are separate. The national bodies responsible are the ACGME and the ABMS, though the latter has no specific authority over the examination of individual candidates. The ABMS only approves new types of certification, including proposals for examination in those new types of certification. The ABMS is more a federation of autonomous boards and, as such, certification in the U.S. has different processes in different specialties. Though there is the impression that standards are reasonably similar, in fact, there are 23 boards and 23 different sets of standards.

The Public Interest

The basic purpose of the certification system is to protect the public interest through the improvement of medical care. This is accomplished through the "setting of professional standards and surveillance of medical qualifications" (Article II of the ABMS Bylaws). The process depends on the judgments of senior, highly respected specialists whose loyalty is to the profession itself and thereby to the health of the citizens. These commitments reflect a different level of concern than the guild interests associated with a union. Such altruism is questioned by critics who suspect that doctors are interested only in their own economic gain. Some have suggested that the public interest is better protected by the state (or some level of government) than by the private sector. Physicians challenge that assumption, pointing to the complications of bureaucracy and politics and the tendency of government to settle for lower rather than higher standards. It has been true in the U.S. licensure system (operated by the government) that minimal standards are adopted for the protection of the public rather than standards of excellence.

Some organizations use the appointment of one or more "public members" to assure input from outside the profession. While the concept of a public member (the ABMS has three and at least two of the ABMS Boards have one or more) has been found useful, it is always a challenge to that person to truly represent the public. Indeed, how can one among 15 professionals, represent the concerns of a very large and diverse public? It would be unusual to find that here was a single point of view from the public. Thus the representative will find it difficult to even know, let alone put forth, the multiple views of the "public."

One problem for the public is to have useful information about the medical specialist and subspecialist system. How can an average citizen understand the functions and qualifications of each type of specialist and how can that citizen find a competent specialist—assuming that the citizen knows which specialist to locate? We have depended on the concept of a primary (personal) physician to be the advocate for the patient—to provide not only continuing and comprehensive care, but to make intelligent use of consultant subspecialists. But does every citizen have a primary physician and can we be assured that those who are such, function efficiently in using the subspecialist system? A challenge for the future is to examine whether the present system is working and in what manner it should be changed if change is required.

Does Subspecialism Enhance the Quality of Care?

The tertiary care system of the western world (especially the U.S. and Canada) is the envy of the rest of the globe. Patients with complex illnesses in the Mid-East, Africa, South America, and Asia, who can afford to do so, come to North America for medical care. In the U.S.A. and Canada it is assumed that quality health care is a right, although there are increasing concerns about the costs of health care, there is equal demand for accessibility and quality. We take it as an article of faith that medical science (and the subspecialism which is its consequence) enhances the quality of care. But, the miracles of medical science that have demonstrably prolonged life, have brought certain complications.

Subspecialization is said to fragment care and though the patient may obtain superior expertise by seeing several specialists, it requires sophistication and remarkable coordination to get to the right experts in the right order. The complications associated with seeing many doctors and the confusion in trying to understand all of their messages have made the myth of the horse-and-buggy doctor (who knew the entire family but could cure few conditions) attractive. The concept of primary care has become very popular, especially among legislators. The primary care physician is the one who is presumed to be the point of first contact, the coordinator of care when it must involve other specialists and subspecialists, and the personal physician who is always available to provide continuity of care. Medicine has seen considerable concern about primary care—defining which physicians are truly primary care specialists and the fact that subspecialists also practice primary care medicine. In the U.S., certain economic advantages make it desirable to have one's specialty defined as a primary care specialty and there has been confusion in this area. Though there is little disagreement that the general internist, general pediatrician and family practitioner are primary care physicians, the obstetrician/gynecologists point out that they provide primary care to a certain population (women) and the psychiatrists take the same position since they deal with a large number of the institutionalized mentally ill as the primary care physician. General surgeons have also been called primary care physicians. The fact that 38% of all internists ever certified in the U.S. also have subspecialty certification (and in this generation, 62% of internists go on to take subspecialty fellowships) does not remove the fact that these subspecialists spend a large proportion of their time doing general internal medicine (primary care). Some have asked if one can maintain skills effectively as both a subspecialist and primary care physician, but that question has not been scientifically tested. Those who question the need for such large numbers of subspecialists suggest that 80-90% of the patients seen by a subspecialist could be treated by a general specialist and ask whether the high degree of subspecialism increases the cost of medical care. Subspecialists are presumed to be willing to see patients with problems in their area of expertise and the availability of subspecialists is said by some to encourage unnecessary referrals to the "expert." The RCPSC adopted a policy statement on primary care in 1983 which pointed to the fact that a number of subspecialists may devote part of their time to primary care and to the Canadian concerns about a definition of who should be considered a primary care specialist. That policy statement reflected discussions spanning a number of years. In the U.S., the ABMS studied the field a few years earlier (1975), but the fact is that these ambiguities about definition of a primary care specialist and concerns about the total professional activities of the primary care physician continue to the present. The joint conference of the ABMS and the RCPSC did not focus on this issue, but it clearly was one of the problems that will continue to be of concern in both countries.

Gatekeepers

Some have suggested that a gatekeeper, preferably the patient's primary care physician, would help avoid fragmentation of care. A gatekeeper would have to be consulted before the patient could receive treatment or consultation from a specialist or subspecialist. Presently, many managed care plans and HMO's require such control—ostensibly to enhance the quality of care through appropriate use of specialists, but actually to contain costs. Most specialty and subspecialty groups resist this suggestion out of the conviction that patients have the right to seek medical care from the physician of their choice, and out of the fear that gatekeepers will lower the quality of care in their zeal to reduce costs. The future is likely to see marked changes, at least in the U.S., and many now predict that 25% of the U.S. population will be served by HMO's and 60% by managed care plans which are likely to use the gatekeeper system. The real struggle will be the effort to maintain quality of care while reducing costs. It has been said that there are no cheap parachutes, fire extinguishers or quality medical specialists.

Hospital Privileges

In the U.S., hospital medical staffs determine what a physician is permitted to do in that particular hospital. Though the governing board of that hospital is legally responsible, such boards are likely to accept the recommendations of their medical staff. Since privileges govern the physician's activities (and his income), they may be a point of contention, because such controls of physician privileges are meant to protect the public and the quality of its care. The determination of privileges has often depended on credentials and, in the U.S., medical staffs are inclined to look at certification in a specialty or subspecialty as an important determinant in awarding privileges. Credentials should not, however, be the sole determinant of privileges. An ABMS statement on delineation of staff privileges states:

> It is recognized that there are various methods for delineating clinical privileges. In making the determination of what privileges a practitioner will be permitted to exercise in a hospital, medical specialty certification or subcertification should be considered as only one of several valid and important criteria. It should be emphasized that there is no specific requirement for a diplomate in a recognized specialty to hold certification in a subspecialty of that field in order to include aspects of that subspecialty within the range of privileges.

In spite of that position, many hospital medical staffs look for a set of national standards to make decisions about privileges and thus avoid the responsibility for making judgments based on performance and competence as well as on credentials. The reality is that each credential tends to offer the possibility of serving as a requirement for certain clinical activities. Credentials may build walls around practices if so used. It has been said that certification and subcertification has become "de facto licensure." Since the certification process evaluates a physician's knowledge, skills and attitudes at a point in time, it cannot always predict future performance. Testing the predictive validity of certification is a challenge that is being explored, but neither the ratings of performance during the residency or on the cross-sectional certification examinations have been proven to constantly predict performance. Even recertification (voluntary or imposed by time-limited certification) cannot offer such guarantees.

The challenge to the delineation of clinical privileges is to rate actual performance in practice. The U.S. specialty boards, in collaboration with other agencies, are discussing new methods of performance-oriented measures and the contribution of the specialty boards may be the development of useful methods of rating performance. It would aid the hospital medical staffs as well as the boards themselves.

The Costs of Subspecialization

The increasing costs of health care are frequently attributed to subspecialty medicine. The additional training is expensive. Specialists are accused of encouraging the use of more tests and procedures than the primary care practitioner. Evaluation by several subspecialists is probably more costly than the use of a single physician. Subspecialists are also said to encourage more surgical procedures. However, there are no studies that readily demonstrate this additional cost when quality is considered. Indeed, it is extremely difficult to do cost/benefit studies without considering the benefit of high-quality medical care. There are many procedures and treatments that require a very high degree of skill and most Americans realize that. While calling for more primary care physicians, the average person will also insist on the highest quality care and a platoon of the most expert physicians available. Such is the value placed on care for one's self or loved ones, though the concerns about costs are very real. Hopefully, the studies will attempt to scientifically test hypotheses about the relationship of quality care to skill and to benefits.

The cost containment efforts in the U.S. have been channeled through a competition approach. The concept that competition replaces regulation in order to drive down costs, has resulted in a market economy. Instead of the traditional solo or small group fee-for-service practice, physicians are increasingly likely to be associated with managed care. Hospitals are even more likely to group together for economy of operation, in joint efforts to compete for patients, and to gain access to capital necessary to deal with today's expensive technology.

Competition in health care leaves questions about the quality of care. The effect of U.S. efforts in establishing a prospective pricing system with Diagnosis Related Group reimbursement has radically altered the concept of Medicare paying for any service medically necessary. Unquestionably it has reduced costs with shorter lengths of stay, fewer hospital admissions, and the past two years have seen hospital bed vacancies and reduced staffs.

Since hospitals have been the major source of funds for the education of specialists and subspecialists, these changes in hospital funding have resulted in a major review of the funding of graduate medical education. As this is written there are several legislative proposals to radically alter the use of U.S. Medicare funds for training specialists. Whatever is finally passed will doubtlessly affect other payers such as U.S. Medicaid, insurance companies, etc. All of these matters will affect the complex system of the education of specialists in the U.S. and will contribute to the confusion about manpower planning, the role of specialist and subspecialists, and the entire system of medical care. Contributing to that complexity is the alleged surplus of physicians. The U.S. GMENAC studies accurately predicted the large increases in numbers of U.S. physicians, including both graduates of U.S. and Canadian schools, and foreign medical graduates. Many areas that formerly lacked specialist physicians (rural and inner city locations) now have them. Hospital medical staffs feel a surplus of some kinds of specialists. Practitioners report keen competition, all of which leads to the conviction that we truly have a "doctor glut" in the U.S. From one point of view a surplus of specialists is assumed to reduce costs, but from another it may also be expensive because physicians tend to create costs in their search for quality medical care.

Subspecialism and Medical Education

Specialization has had a major impact on the education of physicians and the organization of medical schools. Though graduate medical education (residencies and fellowships that provide the education of specialists and subspecialists) is artificially separated from medical schools in the U.S., the two interact very significantly. From the point of view of GME the "student" gives patient care under supervision and learns in the process. The resident or fellow is paid a stipend and the cost of stipends and teaching are generally assumed by hospital patient care funds in the U.S. In medical schools the students pay tuition, give very little direct patient care and the responsibilities are those of the medical school. However, the faculties of both residency programs and medical schools are much the same people—at least in the clinical departments. Medical students are taught by the subspecialists who are their professors and by the residents in those subspecialties. The subspecialists on the faculty become professors because subspecialization is the generally accepted avenue to professorships. The subspecialists have high prestige because they are the most knowledgable and competent in a given area in accordance with the system of values in all fields in the universities. Thus, the most respected teachers and role models are the subspecialists and it is not surprising that enterprising students want to model themselves after their professors and seek similar credentials.

Medical schools feel compelled to have *all* specialties and subspecialties represented on their faculties in order to offer excellence in education and to compete with other medical schools for grants and awards to enhance the scholarship of the school. Even in areas of concentrated populations which have several medical schools it is not customary to regionalize subspecialties or to combine the resources needed to have expensive technologies. The entire system tends to place higher status and rewards in the subspecialist career than the generalist and in today's world, non-specialist careers are rejected by more than 90% of medical students.

All of these factors lead to a system of subspecialty care of high quality, but with problems of cost, manpower numbers and distribution, and organization of the health care delivery system outlined here.

Summary

1. The conference on which this book was based, did not make recommendations or take actions. The purpose was to identify concerns in the U.S. and Canada, two countries with a special relationship. The issues discussed at the conference and in this book will be used by each organization in its own policy and decision-making processes.

2. Though there are concerns about proliferation of subspecialties and the possibilities for fragmentation of care, we cannot stop the development of new subspecialties. Their appearance is inevitable and that is the way it should be. That is part of progress in medical science. Any accommodation to this trend must not weaken the bedrocks and foundations of the primary specialties. The value of identification with one's primary specialty (not necessarily a "primary care" specialty, but the basic specialty in which training took place before any subspecialty training) must be emphasized. The subspecialty certificates *could* tend to erode that and such a tendancy must be avoided.

3. In dealing with this potential fragmentation, the ABMS and the RCPSC should provide leadership and not be regarded as anchors dragging their collective heels and impeding progress. It is the responsibility of both organizations to authorize new forms of certification, a responsibility which requires careful planning and considered action. The ABMS effort in this direction is to develop a new type of certification called "Added Qualifications." The RCPSC is considering initially accrediting new subspecialty training programs using national standards without offering a full certification process. There may be institutional certification for the graduates of such programs in the early years with the possibility of RSPSC certification at a later date. They are not "final answers," but point to the need for continuing concern.

4. A manpower data base is essential to understanding the developments in the role of specialists and subspecialists in the health care system. This does not suggest that planning should control manpower. The U.S. has had its GMENAC and SOSSUS reports, but our experience with government is that it predicts wide swings with resultant inefficiency. During the early 1960s, the U.S. government predicted major shortages and called for doubling the size of MD graduating classes along with immigration preference to attract foreign physicians. Twenty years later we predict a significant oversupply of physicians and propose cutbacks. The ABMS and the RCPSC should not assume responsibility for manpower *planning* but should make available valid data on medical specialists. The RCPSC in cooperation with the CMA and national specialty societies is launching such a project in four specialties. The ABMS has developed an automated data base for biographic data on certified specialists. Those data bases should seek to provide specific data about the FMGs who now constitute 23% of practitioners in the U.S. and Canada. Special concerns about the quality of education in Caribbean medical schools have been raised and must be answered.

5. In the U.S. corporatization of medical care, a shift to competition

instead of regulation, the move away from solo practice on a fee-for-service basis, the entry of nonmedical practitioners into medical practice, and the "physician glut" have created revolutionary changes in less than five years. These changes have affected and will create changes in specialty practice, and therefore the education and certification of specialists. Despite the murkiness of our crystal ball, we must take those changes into account as the leaders of the specialty certification system. In Canada, the changes are somewhat different but no less significant. The RCPSC and ABMS should exchange information and viewpoints about dealing with changes in the health care system.

6. Recertification does not occur in Canada, and it is not universally accepted in the U.S. Nevertheless, seven of the 23 boards have instituted time-limited certification and an eighth is likely to follow suit this year. The rapid rate of change in medical science and the interaction between privileging and certification will put pressure on all specialties to be active in recertification—voluntary or mandatory. Recertification is likely to be more acceptable when it can be done as a performance evaluation rather than total dependance on cognitive tests.

7. Jurisdictional concerns and "turf" disputes will continue and probably be intensified in this period of competition and concern about a surplus of physicians. It is also a consequence of changes in practice and therefore changes in education—both calling for appropriate credentials. The ABMS is presently concerned with credentials in horizontal skills—fields of practice which are common to more than one primary specialty. This motivated the addition of the credential called "Added Qualifications." Whether this will diminish the intensity of jurisditional disputes remains to be seen. Other ways of dealing with "turf" must be found.

Appendix
A Selected and Annotated Bibliography on Specialization

John S. Lloyd, Ph.D.

This appendix contains a bibliography, the references for which were selected and annotated by the author. They represent a mixture of considered opinion and empirical investigation related to the subject of medical specialization and subspecialization. Most of the former references bemoan the intendant fragmentation which accompaines specialization and subspecialization but offer few solutions to counteract the apparent inevitability of continued proliferation of new subspecialties. It is designed to provide background reading for the other, more recent opinions expressed elsewhere in this book.

1966

Bowers RF: Is Superspecialization Harmful? *Surgery,* 60:1120-1122.

Author's answer to the question in the title of this editorial is yes—to the patient. "Superspecialization" is harmful when it restricts the physician's view of the patient to conform to the limited purview of his/her specialty.

1969

Who is a Specialist? *JAMA,* 207:746.

Editorial explaining the roles of ABMS, AMA, and the "Essentials for

Approval of Examining Boards in Medical Specialties" in the recognition of new specialty boards in the U.S.

1970

Menke WG: Divided Labor: The Doctor as Specialist. *Annals of Internal Medicine*, 72:943-950.

Specialization is both a product of and a contributor to the scientific information explosion in medicine. It subdivides both doctor and patient, increases the difficulty of attaining a clear sense of medical identity for students and young physicians, and places additional strain on the traditional doctor-patient relationship. Specialization emphasizes the science of medicine and its rational processes in the treatment of disease and contributes to depersonalization, aggravates patient anxieties, and implicitly encourages quackery. It is probably the major factor disturbing traditional ethical and economic patterns in medicine, and it dominates medical education and research and medical practice, promotes jurisdictional disputes with the profession, and weakens organizational strength and professional power.

1971

Stevens R: *American Medicine and the Public Interest*, New Haven: Yale University Press.

Authoritative account of development of specialization in medicine during the past century and its implications for the cost and organization of medical care and for medical education. Particularly relevant to the present book is Chapter 15, entitled: "Pressures for New Specialty Boards: A Process of Fragmentation."Contains valuable historical perspective on period prior to 1970 regarding the forces promoting and retarding fragmentation of medicine into more and more specialties.

1972

Hanlon CR: Specialization in Medicine. *Journal of Thoracic and Cardiovascular Surgery*, 64:179-185.

Traces the history of specialization in medicine from ancient to modern times. Asserts that surgical privileges should be given only to "those with recognized credentials and demonstrated competence"; points out the contradiction in calling family (general) practice a specialty; and chides the specialties over their internecine jurisdictional squabbles rather than uniting to battle the encroachment of government bureaucracy and those who would manage medicine as an industry.

1973

Eckert C: Specialization and Superspecialization in Surgery. *Archives of Surgery,* 109:139-142.

Presidential address presented at about the time that pediatric surgery was to become the *first area* to be awarded a certificate of special qualification under the American Board of Surgery. The author warns that other subspecialty areas (e.g., vascular surgery, critical care medicine, hand surgery) were waiting in the wings to be recognized. He argues against further fragmentation of general surgery which would result from these other areas becoming recognized by certificates of special qualification.

Beck JC: Certification and the Specialty Board. *Bulletin of New York Academy of Medicine,* 50:1222-1227.

Addresses the question: Who should certify competence in a specialty in the U.S.A.? In answer, author explores pros and cons of a variety of entities and options, including universities and medical schools, hospitals, specialty societies, AMA, federal government and NBME. Option author favors is specialty boards and ABMS.

Longmire WP: Who is to Certify Competence in a Specialty? *Bulletin of New York Academy of Medicine,* 50:1228-1230.

Addresses the question: Who should certify competence in a specialty in the U.S.A.? Present system of specialty boards works quite well. Certification by such a voluntary, self-sustaining apparatus could be strengthened by restricting hospital specialty privileges to certified specialists, by paying certified specialists more than uncertified specialists for the same services, and by federal or state laws regulating specialty practice.

1974

Redlich FC: The Specialty Boards and Standards of Competence. *Bulletin of New York Academy of Medicine,* 50:1231-1234.

Addresses the question: Who should certify competence in a specialty in the U.S.A.? Specialty boards are only one of a variety of professional and public controls on medical competence. Author reviews frequent criticisms of specialty boards. Concludes that the positive and constructive contributions of voluntary certifying boards toward raising standards of medical competence has been far greater than the negative impact implied in the criticisms.

1975

Chase RA: Proliferation of Certification in Medical Specialties: Productive or Counterproductive. *New England Journal of Medicine,* 294:497-499.

Argues that continued proliferation of different forms of certification in medical specialties may be counterproductive to quality of and accessibility to health care. Certification must not carry with it an exclusive right to practice in that specialty. Solution proposed is better health care delivery system planning and organization at local or regional level.

1976

Petersdorf RG: Internal Medicine 1976: Consequences of Subspecialization and Technology. *Annals of Internal Medicine,* 84:92-94.

Discusses the effect of subspecialization and technology on the general internist. Both appear to increase cost and risk as well as to produce fragmented and often inhumane care. General internists should be major providers of primary care to adults.

Varco RL: Fragmentation in Medicine: Continuing Proliferation in Varieties of Certificates of Special Competence. *Human Pathology,* 7:1-2.

Describes the disadvantages of the proliferation of certificates of special competence (now qualification) under the aegis of specialty boards and the ABMS. Urges far more stringent process of evaluating new applications for issuing such certificates.

1979

Aiken LH, et al: The Contribution of Specialists to the Delivery of Primary Care: A New Perspective. *New England Journal of Medicine,* 300:1363-1370.

Two national studies have shown that one of every five Americans now receives continuing general medical care from a specialist physician. Our study suggests that, despite the current shortage of generalist-physician services, continuing specialist participation in primary care will lead to sufficient generalist medical services by the mid-1980s. Whether specialist participation is the most appropriate or cost-effective way to improve access to such care is unclear. However, until this question is resolved, more governmental regulation of graduate medical education may be unwise. Offering all physicians, regardless of specialty, more primary-care experience during residency training might better deal with this aspect of American medical practice.

See also related editorial in same issue: Relman AS: Generalists and Specialists. pp. 1386-1387.

Luce JM, Byyny RL: The Evolution of Medical Specialism. *Perspectives in Biology and Medicine,* 22:377-389.

Traces history of medical specialization from ancient to modern times (the latter in U.S.A.). Specialism did not evolve from generalism, rather specialism preceded generalism. Specialism is a result of social, environmental and technological factors as well as the desires of the medical profession. Today's emphasis on primary care specialties is a return to generalism—perhaps the first time that the balance between the number of generalists and specialists has been planned to meet the needs of health care delivery in the U.S.A.

1980

Beeson PB: The Natural History of Medical Subspecialties. *Annals of Internal Medicine,* 93:624-626.

Factors that have favored the division of the field of internal medicine into numerous subspecialties during the past three decades are reviewed. Some specialty areas are suited almost exclusively to academic clinical investigators, whereas others can be the basis for private practice. Some requisites for viability as a practice subspecialty are listed. It is suggested that in the coming decade the pendulum of preference is likely to swing back somewhat, with a larger fraction of young internists choosing to be identified as practicing general internal medicine rather than limiting their work to a single subspecialty.

Rogers DE, Aiken LH: General Medical Care in America: A Generalist-Specialist Mix. *American Journal of Medicine,* 68:160-162.

Cites data from recent studies indicating that general medical care in the U.S. is not only provided by generalists but also by specialists. Whether the quality of general medical care was the same in both groups of patients was not known.

Stevens R: The Changing Ideas of a Medical Specialty. *Transactions [Studies of the College of Physicians of Philadelphia,* 5:159-177.

Traces changes in the idea or meaning or perception of specialization during the last century. Originally, to be specialized meant to add to the capabilities of a general physician, thus broadening his/her scope. As specialization became institutionalized it became associated with "scientific conservatism" and narrowness of interest and practice. Geriatrics is examined in light of the evolving meanings of a specialty.

1981

Longmire WP: Changing Patterns of Surgical Training and Practice. *American Journal of Surgery,* 141:632-637.

"Personal reflections" on surgical training, manpower, practice and research, and the roles of specialty societies, specialty boards and the government in regard to these subjects.

Rhee SO, et al: Domain of Practice and the Quality of Physician Performance. *Medical Care,* 19:14-23.

This study has attempted to determine the relationship between physician domain of practice and their quality of medical care. The study examined whether there was a quality difference in practice either 1) between general practitioners and specialists, or 2) between specialists practicing within and outside their specialty domains. The sample consisted of 454 physicians of Hawaii, involving 18 specialty categories: general practitioners (133) and specialists (321). The study finds that when the general practitioners . . . practiced without limitation; their quality of care was not as good as that of the specialists. The study also found that when the specialists practiced outside their specialty areas, the relative quality of their performance declined. The latter finding was sustained even when other important practice and background variable were held constant.

1982

Gonnella JS, Veloski JJ: The Impact of Early Specialization on the Clinical Competence of Residents. *New England Journal of Medicine*, 306:275-277.

To study the relation between first-year postgraduate training and performance on a test of general clinical competence, we analyzed results on the Part III National Board Examination according to the type of residency chosen by 1514 graduates of Jefferson Medical College between 1970 and 1979. The results show that physicians in family medicine, internal medicine, or flexible programs score higher on Part III than do those in surgery, pediatrics, obstetrics/gynecology, psychiatry, or pathology, even after correction for their performance on Part II of the boards. Although these differences could be due to other factors, we suggest that in the first year of some residency programs, knowledge and skills in broad areas of medicine are not being sufficiently emphasized, and that changes are needed to strengthen the residents' general capabilities. (See also letters to the editor of same journal with same title; 307:107-108).

Gritzer G: Occupational Specialization in Medicine: Knowledge and Market Explanations. In Roth, J.A. (Ed.) *Research in the Sociology of Health Care. Volume 2: Changing Structure of Health Service Occupations. Greenwich*, CT: JAI Press.

Sociological analysis of specialization in medicine and allied health. Examines development of orthopaedic surgery, rehabilitation medicine, radiology, physical therapy, and corrective therapy to show that control over market segments outweighs the evolution and expansion of knowledge in the drive toward specialization.

Julian OC: Certification of Peripheral Vascular Surgeons. *Annals of Thoracic Surgery*, 33:114-115.

Summarizes problems encountered in bringing order to the field of peripheral vascular surgery as well as potential mechanisms to solve them.

See also related letter to editor of same journal: Mulder, DG Certification of Vascular Surgeons, pp. 304-305.

Smith RJ: Subcertification for Hand Surgery. *Journal of Hand Surgery*, 7:107-112.

Arguments presented in favor of subcertification in hand surgery. Also presents brief history of development of specialization in Europe and

U.S. Emphasis on role of specialty societies and specialty boards in formation of specialties and subspecialties during twentieth century.

Spencer FC: Thoracic Surgeons and Vascular Surgery. *Annals of Thoracic Surgery,* 33:107-113.

Traces historical development of vascular surgery as a subspecialty and the implication of that development for general surgery and thoracic surgery. Need to find mechanism for accreditation of fellowships as well as the hazards of certification of special qualifications by the American Board of Surgery are discussed.

1983

ACS Statement on Training and Certification. *Bulletin of American College of Surgeons,* 68:72.

"Special areas of interest and training within the recognized surgical specialties . . . should not be recognized by formal certification or by issuance of a certificate of special competence by a specialty board or by an accrediting body."

Bates RC: My Specialty is Doomed. *Medical Economics,* 60:101-111.

Predicts the eventual extinction of the general internist brought on by the erosion of general internal medicine by its own subspecialties as well as by the emergence of family practice as a specialty.

Davidson RA: Birds, Fish, and Subspecialists: A Common Pathway to Extinction. *JAMA,* 250:1386.

Subspecialization may lead to extinction. Medicine and society should put as much value on the generalist who is expert at "comprehensive thinking" as they do on specialization.

Longmire WP: Surgical Turf or Who Should Do What to Whom? *Surgery, Gynecology [Obstetrics,* 156:76-78.

Describes the "laissez-faire" posture of American surgery to the definition of boundaries between surgical specialties and subspecialties. Suggests the need for a consensus definition of areas of jurisdiction so as to improve training and patient care. "Is it possible to divide the turf in order to know who is qualified to do what to whom?"

Vladutiu AO: Cut Down Proliferation of Medical Specialty Certifications. *JAMA,* 250:2284.

This letter decrying "malignant proliferation of certifications" was instigated by the authorization for the American Boards of Allergy & Immunology, Internal Medicine, Pathology, and Pediatrics to issue certificates of special qualification in laboratory immunology in March, 1983. "What is the rationale for so many boards and certifications in one of the laboratory fields? Do those who practice laboratory immunology need certifications (from the many to choose from) to keep their jobs?"

1984

Adamson GD, Rowe HE: Certification of Specialists: Survey of Candidates and Review of the Literature. *Canadian Medical Association Journal*, 130:586-590.

To evaluate the specialty certification process, the Canadian Association of Internes and Residents (CAIR) surveyed 634 candidates who had attempted the written and oral exams of the Royal College of Physicians and Surgeons of Canada. The results suggest that in-training evaluation is a more reliable and valid assessment of competence than the written and oral exams. There is a lack of well defined program objectives that are coordinated with the examinations. CAIR recommends that the present concept of an examination "hurdle" be replaced by different, integrated methods of assessment during training, and that an effective appeal mechanism be developed.

Ell SR: Five Hundred Years of Specialty Certification and Compulsory Continuing Medical Education. *JAMA*, 251:752-753.

From 1300 to 1801, Venice required an early form of specialty certification for medical practice and the yearly attendance of refresher courses in anatomy by all licensed practitioners in the city. The latter requirement provoked ingenious evasions, which the Venetian government continually tried to overcome. This article describes the system and its implementation, based on Venetian archival documents.

King LS: Medical Practice: Specialization. *JAMA*, 251:1333-1338.

Discussion of emergence of specialization during latter half of 19th century in U.S., factors contributing to this emergence, and the resultant tension it created between general practitioners and specialists. Particular emphasis on role of AMA in this process.

Perler BA, Zuidema GD: The Effect of Vascular Fellowships on General Surgical Residency Training. *Annals of Surgery*, 200:247-254.

To answer the controversial question of whether or not vascular fellowships detract from general surgical training, questionnaires were sent to directors of 41 approved vascular fellowship programs, 41 residency directors in the same institutions, and 40 residency directors in unversity programs without approved fellowships. Overall response rate was 74% (93% of vascular fellowship directors, 63% of same-institution residency directors, and 65% of residency directors without vascular fellowships). Thirty-four percent of fellowship directors and 38% of same-institution residency directors indicated that the fellowship has reduced the vascular surgery case load of residents. In institutions with fellowships, general surgery residents performed an average of 71 major vascular procedures and first assisted on 44, whereas residents performed 65 major vascular procedures and assisted on 47 in institutions without fellowships. Overall, 79% of fellowship directors and 62% of same-institution general surgical directors indicated that the fellowship improved the quality of vascular surgical training. Only 15% of same-institution residency directors and 3% of fellowship directors felt that the fellowship detracted from the general surgical experience. Fifteen per cent of institutions without approved fellowships have now initiated vascular fellowship programs, and an additional 23% plan to begin such fellowships. No fellowship directors plan to abolish their programs, although 8% plan to decrease the number of fellows in order to increase general surgery resident participation. Among the majority of institutions studied, vascular fellowships have not adversely affected general surgical training, and often enhanced it.

1985

Shephard DAE: Certification of Medical Specialists in Canada, 1934-1984: A Half-Century of Progress. *Annals RCPSC*, 18:44-48.

Although the certification of medical and surgical specialists is centuries old—it is essentially a 20th-century aspect of professionalization. In Canada, the body that certifies specialists is The Royal College of Physicians and Surgeons of Canada, which was founded in 1929. The Royal College first became concerned with certification in 1934, when it was asked by the College of Physicians and Surgeons of Saskatchewan to advise on the use of the term "specialist." Over the years, interest in certification has continued unabated. The half-century that elapsed since 1934 closed with the publication in 1984 of a somewhat out of date but nonetheless challenging study by the Canadian Association of Internes and Residents (see Adamson & Rowe above). At the end of this half-century, it is appropriate to trace the evolution of the certification program in Canada and to comment on it.

1985

Wassersug JD: Subspecialists Are Squeezing Me Out. *Medical Economics,* 62:65.

A general internist bemoans the fact that his patients demand they be seen by subspecialists for all but the most minor illnesses.

Appendix

Contributors

John A. Benson, Jr., M.D.
American Board of Internal Medicine
200 S.W. Market Street, #1930
Portland, OR 97201

Dr. Jean G. Couture
Department of Surgery
1050, Chemin Ste-Foy
Quebec, Que, Canada G1S 4L8

William J. Digman, M.D.
UCLA School of Medicine
Department of Obstetrics/Gynecology
Los Angeles, CA 90024

Dr. Fred DuVal
1502 Medical Arts Building
233 Kennedy Street—Winnipeg
Manitoba, Canada R3C 3J5

Dr. John H. Duff
University Hospital
339 Windemere Road
London, Ont., Canada N6A 5A5

Melvin A. Glasser
Health Action Security Council
1757 N Street, N.W.
Washington, DC 20036

Dr. Ramsay W. Gunton
Department of Medicine
University Hospital
London, Ont., Canada N6A 5A5

C. Rollins Hanlon, M.D.
American College of Surgeons
55 East Erie Street
Chicago, IL 60611

Dr. James E. Hickey
170-172 Fitzroy Street
Charlottetown, P.E.I.
Canada C1A 1S2

Dr. Charles H. Hollenberg
RM 216, Simcoe Hall
27 King's College Circle
Toronto, Ont., Canada M5S 1A1

B. Leslie Huffman, Jr., M.D.
Deepwater Farm
21383 State Rte. 65
Grand Rapids, OH 43522

Robert B. King, M.D.
SUNY—Upstate Medical Center
750 East Adams Street
Syracuse, NY 13210

Kenneth L. Krabbenhoft, M.D.
Department of Radiology
4201 St. Antoine
Detroit, MI 48201

Dr. G. Ross Langley
Suite 8-024
Victoria General Hospital
Halifax, Nova Scotia B3H 2Y9

William E. Laupus, M.D.
East Carolina University
School of Medicine
Greenville, NC 27834

Dr. Carroll A. Laurin
Dept. Orthopaedic Surgery
687 Pine Avenue West
Montreal, Quebec H3A 1A1

Henry J. Mankin, M.D.
Department of Orthopaedic Surgery
Massachusetts General Hospital
Boston, MA 02114

Dr. Lionel E. McLeod
1200 Oxford Tower
10235 - 101 Street
Edmonton, Alberta T5J 3G1

Dr. Yves Morin
11 Cote Du Palais
Quebec, Quebec,
Canada G1R 2J6

Thomas K. Oliver, Jr., M.D.
Children's Hospital
125 Desoto Street
Pittsburgh, PA 15213

Dr. Bernard J. Perey
Victoria General Hospital
Centennial Wing, Suite 8-028
Halifax, Nova Scotia B3H 2Y9

Richard J. Reitemeier, M.D.
Mayo Clinic
200 First Street, SW
Rochester, MN 55905

Arnold S. Relman, M.D., Editor
The New England Journal of Medicine
10 Shattuck Street
Boston, MA 02115

Dr. W.B. Spaulding
1200 Main Street West
Hamilton, Ontario
Canada L8S 4J9

Bruce E. Spivey, M.D.
Pacific Medical Center
Box 7999
San Francisco, CA 94120

Dr. Donald R. Wilson
Hannah Inst., Suite 101
14 Prince Arthur Avenue
Toronto, Ont., Canada M5R 1A9

Participants

Murray R. Abell, M.D., Ph.D.
Edward R. Ames, D.V.M., Ph.D.
Dr. Lee Anolt
James F. Arens, M.D.
Jeanne Arnold, M.D.
Dr. Agnes J. Bishop
Linda L. Blank
Dr. Ian Bowmer
Patrick Bray, M.D.
Dr. Keith Brownell
Robert C. Brownlee, M.D.
Dr. John Burgess
Richard Campbell, M.D.
Richard M. Carter
Mrs. Jo Cassie
Susan Smith Caulk, C.R.N.A.
James Chambers
Mr. Joe Choinard
C. Donald Christian, M.D.
B. Stanley Cohen, M.D.
Dr. Peter J.E. Cruse
Dr. James H. Darragh
Steven J. Davidson, M.D.'
Robert A. Davis
Thomas L. Dent, M.D.
Robert C. Derbyshire, M.D.
Dr. Luc Beschenes
Dr. Henry B. Dinsdale
Steven M. Downing, Ph.D.
Nancy Dyke
Bernard Ferguson
Thomas B. Ferguson, M.D.
Dr. Murray M. Fraser
John C. Gienapp, M.D.
Dr. George Goldsand
Dr. R. Gourdeau
Thorne Griscom, M.D.
Paul L. Grover, Ph.D.
Dr. Ian Hart
Herbert Hohn, M.D.
Dr. Brian Holmes
William J. Horgan, C.C.P.
Dr. C. Stuart Houston
Stephen J. Jay, M.D.
Minu Kashef, M.D.
Eugene L. Ketchum Ph.D.
Samuel Kling, M.D.
Joan E. Knapp
Thomas J. Krizek, M.D.
Donald G. Langsley, M.D.
Dr. Francois Laramee
Pierrette Leonard
Clarence S. Livingood, M.D.
John S. Lloyd, Ph.D.
Dr. Jean-Marie Loiselle
Dr. J.A. Low
Dr. Frederick Lowy
Dr. S. Clair MacLeod
M. Stephen Mahaley, Jr., M.D.
Dr. Michel V. Mathieu
William E. Matory, M.D.
Dr. Robert Maudsley
Brian F. McCabe, M.D.
Dr. J.D. McCallum
Jean McDaniel
Dr. D.M. McDougal
Glen McStavick
John L. Melvin, M.D.
James A Merrill, M.D.
Steven E. Minnick, M.D.
Benson S. Munger, Ph.D.
Dr. David A. Murphy
Nancie Noie
Louise Papineau
Dr. R. Patey
Dr. William M. Paul
Dr. Graham Pineo
Nicholas J. Pisacano, M.D.

Dr. Gerard E. Plante
George Podgorny, M.D.
Bertram A. Portin, M.D.
George F. Reed, M.D.
Dr. Donald Rice
Dr. Jean Rochon
Richard H. Sanders, P.C.
Dr. Robert Sheppard
Ben Shimberg
Dr. D.P. Snidal
Dr. Brian J. Sproule
Mrs. Ruth Stockdale
I.H. Strasburger, M.D.
Dr. DeGuise Vaillancourt
John A. Van Buskirk, M.D.
Dr. John Wade
David K. Wagner, M.D.
Alexander J. Walt, M.D.
Mrs. Sheila Waugh
Peyton Weary, M.D.
Robert B. Welch, M.D.
John G. Wiegenstein, M.D.

Index

Q

R

S

ragh, M.D.

h is its consequence) enhances the quality of
lical science that have demonstrably prolonged
omplications.
o fragment care and though the patient may
seeing several specialists, it requires sophisti-
lination to get to the right experts in the right
ociated with seeing many doctors and the con-
nd all of their messages have made the myth
or (who knew the entire family but could cure
The concept of primary care has become very
egislators. The primary care physician is the
the point of first contact, the coordinator of
ner specialists and subspecialists, and the per-
available to provide continuity of care. Medi-
concern about primary care defining which
care specialists and the fact that subspecialists
edicine. In the U.S., certain economic advan-
one's specialty defined as a primary care
confusion in this area. Though there is little
internist, general pediatrician and family prac-
ysicians, the obstetrician-gynecologists point
ry care to a certain population (women) and
e position since they deal with a large number
ally ill as the primary care physician. General
d primary care physicians. The fact that 38%
in the U.S. also have subspecialty certifica-
62% of internists go on to subspecialty
the fact that these subspecialists spend a large
ng general internal medicine (primary care).
maintain skills effectively as both a sub-
physician, but that question has been seri-
question the need for such large numbers of
0-90% of the patients seen by a subspecialist
l specialist and ask whether the high degree
the cost of medical care. Subspecialists are
patients with problems in the area of exper-
subspecialists is said by
"expert." The R
83 which point
part of their tim
in on of wh

mary care specialist. That policy statement re[illegible] a number of years. In the U.S., the ABMS stat[illegible] earlier (1975), but the fact is that these ambig[illegible] a primary care specialist and concerns about the[illegible] ties of the primary care physician continue to [illegible] ference of the ABMS and the RCPSC did not [illegible] clearly was one of the problems that will con[illegible] both countries.

Gatekeepers

Some have suggested that a gatekeeper, prefera[illegible] care physician, would help avoid fragmentatio[illegible] would have to be consulted before the patient c[illegible] consultation from a specialist or subspecialist. [illegible] care plans and HMO's require such control—[illegible] quality of care through appropriate use of special[illegible] costs. Most specialty and subspecialty groups [illegible] of the conviction that patients have the right t[illegible] the physician of their choice, and out of the [illegible] lower the quality of care in their zeal to reduce [illegible] to see marked changes, at least in the U.S., an[illegible] 25% of the U.S. population will be served by HM[illegible] care plans which are likely to use the gatekeeper [illegible] will be the effort to [illegible] in quality of care w[illegible] been said that there are [illegible] cheap parachutes, fir[illegible] medical specialists.

Hospital Privileges

In the U.S., hospital medical staffs determine wh[illegible] to do in that particular hospital. Though the gov[illegible] tal is legally responsible, such boards are likely t[illegible] tions of their medical staff. Since privileges gover[illegible] (and his income), they may be a point of conte[illegible] trols of physician privileges are meant to protect [illegible] of its care. The determination of privileges has c[illegible] tials [illegible] in the U.S. medical staffs are inclin[illegible] in [illegible] ty or subspecialty as an important [illegible] priv[illegible] edentials should not, however, b[illegible] [illegible] an ABMS statement or delineation